THE POWER PRINCIPLE:
Mind-Body-Spirit Approach to Ultimate Weight Loss

Sergey Sorin, MD

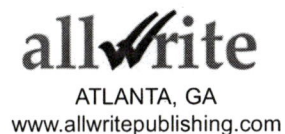

ATLANTA, GA
www.allwritepublishing.com

Copyright © August 2008 by Sergey Sorin.

All rights reserved. No part of this publication may be reproduced, stored in a retrieval system, or transmitted in any form or by any means, electronic, mechanical, photocopying, recording or otherwise, without the prior written permission of the copyright owner.

Although every effort was made to ensure the accuracy and completeness of information contained in this book, we assume no responsibility for errors, inaccuracies, omissions, or inconsistency herein. The information in this book is provided for your general purposes only. It does not constitute personal medical advice, and you should consult your own physician if you have any questions or concerns about any information in this book or before pursuing any course of treatment.

For more information, contact the publisher:
Allwrite Publishing
P.O. Box 1071, Atlanta, GA 30301

Library of Congress Card Catalogue Number: 2008932789
ISBN: 978-0-9744935-5-8

Printed in the United States of America

Cover design by Michael Allen

DEDICATION

Special thanks to my wife, Rosemary, who has been my beautiful angel and my best friend ever since our first meeting. My grandparents, Yakov and Polina, who laid the foundation upon which our entire family has been based and who allowed further generations to stand strong. It's been said that in gaining our accomplishments, we stand upon the shoulders of giants. They are truly the giants in my life and will always be on my mind and in my heart. My mom, Anna, who has given and continues to give me unconditional love and support, overcoming all kinds of obstacles and allowing me to become the person I am now. Also, thanks to my friends and family who stood by me during good times, as well as the hard times. Last but not least, my ultimate and eternal gratitude to the higher power that nurtures me and gives me the strength and motivation to continue my journey both physically and spiritually.

CONTENTS

Foreword, vii

Preface, ix

The "Power of You" Principle 17

PART I: SPIRIT

Chapter 1: Life's Driving Force 21
Personal Worksheet for Discovering the Power of You 26

PART II: MIND

Chapter 2: Intrapersonal Development: Getting on the Right Track 29
Mental States that Affect Weight Control 31
The First, Lasting Steps Toward Success 35
Personal Worksheet for Intrapersonal Development 41
Chapter 3: Interpersonal Development: Dealing with the Outside World 43
Personal Worksheet for Interpersonal Development 48

PART III: BODY

Chapter 4: General Principles for Safe and Effective Dieting 51
Common Types of Diets 52
Counting Calories vs. the Exchange System 54
Types of Diets to Avoid 54
Personal Worksheet for Diet Plans 57
Chapter 5: Recommended Adult Diet Plans 59
High Protein Diets 59
Balanced Low Calorie Diets 62
Personal Worksheet for Adopting a Diet Plan 63
Chapter 6: Weight Loss for Children and Adolescents 65
Personal Worksheet for Parents of Overweight Children and Adolescents .71
Chapter 7: Activity and Exercise 73
Personal Worksheet for Activity and Exercise 81
Chapter 8: Medical History and Weight Gain 83
Personal Worksheets for Medications and Medical Problems 89
Chapter 9: Weight Loss Medications 91
Personal Worksheet for Weight Loss Medications 95
Chapter 10: Weight Loss Surgery 97
Preparing for Surgery 98
Types of Surgeries 98
Personal Worksheet for Weight Loss Surgery 101

Chapter 11: Maintaining Your Progress 103
        Recommendations for Adults 104
        Recommendations for Children and Adolescents 106
        Average Maintenance Needs for Children 108
        Personal Worksheets for Weight Loss Maintenance 109

PART IV: MIND-BODY-SPIRIT

Chapter 12: Power Principle Summary 111

Appendices:
A. Terms Related to Energy (Calorie) Expenditure 117
B. Diet and Nutrition Basics 119
    -Macro-nutrients: Proteins, Carbohydrates, Fats, Alcohol 119
    -Micro-nutrients: Vitamins and Minerals 124
    -Water 126
C. Body Mass Index (BMI) 127
D. Children and Adolescents Weight Percentage Graphs 131
E. Pedometer Weekly Log 136
F. Sample Daily Food/Exercise Planner 137
G. Suggested Adult High Protein, Low Carbohydrate, Low Fat Diet Plans 138
H. Suggested Adult Balanced Diet Plans 144
I. Suggested Adult Maintenance Plans 153
J. Suggested Children and Adolescents Diet Plans 170
K. Suggested Children and Adolescents Maintenance Plans 174
L. Choosing a Medical Weight Loss Program 186

References and Resources 188

FOREWORD

Our country is facing a deadly epidemic, and many doctors are either inept or uninterested in helping its victims overcome the devastating results. The disease is obesity, and it is estimated to be responsible for up to 400,000 excess deaths per year in America. According to recent reports, more than two-thirds of American adults are overweight or obese, and the incidence has been steadily increasing for several years. Clearly, something must be done.

Weight loss is a topic that books, magazines, TV and the Internet frequently address. Yet, many overweight individuals struggle to find a solution that will work for them. They jump from one fad diet to another but never seem to fulfill the promise of hope from the latest "miracle" diet or supplement.

One reason is that obesity is not a "one-size-fits-all" disease. Treatment must be individualized to meet specific needs or it is doomed to fail. The diet that works for Sally may fail miserably for Sue. John is bored with walking for exercise but loves to ride a bike. Mary needs medication for a thyroid condition, and Jill needs one for high insulin levels. Unless the individuality of their "likes" and "needs" is taken into account, a weight loss plan will likely fail.

Most weight loss programs emphasize diet while paying lip service to the role of exercise. Some do the reverse. A few address the need for psychological/behavioral changes. Even fewer dare address "spiritual" factors of importance.

Dr. Sergey Sorin puts it all together in "The Power Principle: Mind-Body-Spirit Approach to Ultimate Weight Loss." Successful weight management involves all three levels: physical, mental and spiritual. Like a 3-legged stool, removing one leg renders it ineffective.

Leaving one ingredient out of a recipe, even if adding an extra amount of another, will have disastrous consequences. That is why a book like this is necessary. It brings all the critical ingredients together, simply explained, in one easily readable book.

Dr. Sorin wisely gives you the tools to individualize your efforts to meet your specific needs. He enlists the best of allies…YOU! Do not gloss over the assignments he asks you to complete. They are an extremely important part of your program.

I suggest you read the book in its entirety to get the big picture. Then re-read it and complete the questionnaires. Most people will benefit greatly from reviewing Part I and Part II frequently, for these are the secret jewels of the book. Come back to them anytime you plateau or are having a difficult time sticking to your program.

Finally, an understanding and knowledgeable bariatric specialist, such as Dr. Sorin, can help you on your journey. Many doctors aren't that interested or trained in this field, but here is one who is. Dr. Sorin even includes information and tips to help you find a specialist who can help you.

It is said that knowledge is power. Dr. Sorin has given you valuable knowledge and tools to empower you to success. If you will add your personal commitment and be persistent, you will not fail.

Michael Steelman, MD, FASBP
Oklahoma City, Oklahoma

PREFACE

Having been born in the former Soviet Union, my family and I experienced what many immigrants from Eastern Europe came to know and ultimately reject – communism. Looking back at my life in the former Soviet Union, up to about the age of 12, I lived in relative poverty with many hardships. Three generations were living in small, congested quarters, which made for lack of personal space, but at the same time, this taught me the value of having a close-knit family and strong family values.

Having grown up in the communist era, significant aspects of social life stand out in stark contrast to my life in the United States. Many cultural and social customs were controlled and restricted as compared to the Western world. One such aspect was related to spirituality—or the lack of it. Any relation or even a slight mention of a higher power other than the communist regime was strictly prohibited. I specifically remember being sent into the "penalty corner" and the school principal for inquiring about such topics. Soon, like many of my peers and family members, I learned not to ask, talk about or even think about certain topics like spirituality. It is quite amazing just how much people can adapt and survive in almost any environment, no matter the atmosphere.

Coming to the United States brought many changes, freedoms and questions. All of a sudden, I had the freedom to think, the freedom to talk and the freedom to act. While "freedom" is a relative term, it was an exciting new concept to embrace for me. Meanwhile, I quickly learned that freedom comes with a price. Having freedom meant having options and having to make decisions that carried potentially limitless lifetime consequences. Along with cultural adjustments came many questions that now had to be addressed, including: who am I; what am I; what do I need; what do I want; and what am I going to do with my life.

My initial search for fulfillment and purpose took me on a path of what is commonly referred to as "The American Dream." After the initial challenge of learning the language, the culture and to do well in school, as well as working part time to help support the family, I made the decision to pursue medicine as a career. After a typical long journey through pre-medical education, medical school, and subsequent training, I took my first job as a physician, which carried with it a notion of relative financial security, status and material possessions. I traveled around the world as much as possible doing missionary and other volunteer work. On top of that, I also tried not only to undertake but also to move beyond typical human adventures. This quest led me to take up scuba diving, skydiving and a wide range of activities. With each new experience and travel, I learned more about myself in the context of the different cultures and circumstances. Nevertheless, the calling for the ultimate meaning and purpose was still as elusive as ever. In retrospect, all the above activities had one thing in common: an outside powerful source was involved.

Despite the relative material success and security from my career and the excitement of my travels, something was missing in my life. I was doing things without understanding why and for what purpose. I was practicing medicine and helping people, but I still did not feel the greater purpose or meaning. I started to identify myself by what I did for a living as a physician. When the job was going well, I felt well; when any question or problem emerged in my professional world, it affected me deeply as well. My family suddenly came back into focus with the illness and death of both of my grandparents. With this, all the insecurities, fears and worries about life, health and death came into perspective. This became the lowest point of my adult life. As a result, my personal, professional and other aspects of life suffered greatly.

However, this was also the turning point and beginning of what would become my personal "enlightenment." I started again from the basics of what this life is all about, its meaning and purpose. This time the focus was no longer on Sergey Sorin, MD, but instead on Sergey, an individual, a part of the universe and my relationship to the higher power and being. A deeper awareness of who I truly am started to emerge.

In the process, I have benefited greatly from reading many literary works and self-help books. I also took great interest and conducted significant personal research into the great spiritual teachings and wisdom within the current and past religious systems, including Western (Judaism, Christianity), as well as Eastern (Hinduism, Buddhism, Taoism, and others). Of particular interest was the mystical component of each of the major spiritual traditions, which emphasize the direct relationship of the individual to a higher purpose. In the process of learning, I tried to focus more on the similarities and basic principles rather than on particular details and customs of each religion.

Being of an analytical, as well as metaphysical, oriented mind and with my training as a physician, I always had questions about the higher power, purpose and reasons. I had an intellectual search for contentment and happiness, as well as for a special feeling or place where everything just made sense. However, a pattern started to appear. The more questions I asked, the less answers took a permanent and lasting stage. Thus, pure intellectual and human reasoning alone was also insufficient.

At that time, I also started learning and participating in meditation (with a higher purpose), a practice that I learned from and will be forever indebted to my friends and colleagues who introduced me to it and continue to serve as mentors and good friends. This was a beginning of a true awakening. This time the focus was on direct experience and connection with the higher power. This felt right, and while some questions remained, the focus shifted from dwelling on the metaphysical to being present in the moment and on experiencing rather than explaining.

It was shortly after this that I experienced another life-changing event, a diagnosis of cancer. When something like this happens to people who are in the prime of their personal and professional lives, the usual response that I have encountered among my own patients involves them going through several systematic stages, including, but not limited to denial, fear, apprehension, anger, and perhaps, at some point, acceptance. Yet, for me, something just instantly clicked following a brief initial adjustment period. I had no fear, no worries, and no regrets, so I had no need to go through the phases. I felt comfort, tranquility, strength, and happiness despite the physical pain, the loss of income, the uncertainty of the future, and possible recurrence. The words and practice of meditation, or in other words, prayer, crystallized faith in my mind, heart and soul.

During that time, I opened my eyes, and I saw my true nature. I am a soul and a spirit who is one with the higher power at the very core. The words I've been saying over and over took meaning. I truly understood and experienced that the outcome is unimportant; what matters is only my best effort. This physical body is only temporary and finite. Thus, it does not define me and neither do any material possessions.

My physical being is a vessel, or in other words, a temple in the service of the higher purpose. It is a temple that I am responsible for maintaining with my very best effort. For without this physical entity, my capacity in this physical world is limited, as I am here for a purpose. Each new day gives me an opportunity to help someone or perhaps many, such as by writing this book. I must take care of my family and friends, as well as strangers who cross my path. I must be good to myself, enjoy life to the fullest, and partake in the beauty that is present, no matter what is happening.

Some other realizations that came as a result of this inward exploration included the capacity to let go of the past, any grudges, regrets, and disappointments. It is still wise to be aware of the past as a predictor and precaution of the future. With knowledge of what *can* happen based on the past, we can better prepare for the present because human nature can take us on a path of good or evil at any given moment. Nonetheless, I made a conscious decision to clear my mind and make the best of the present moment. When we fill our time and energy with self-pity, self-loathing, guilt, anger, hate, and any other negative emotions, we leave no room to experience the most beneficial moments of our lives. When we make a true effort to dispel the negative and harvest the positive, we experience more beauty, happiness, satisfaction and peace.

After my experience with a life-threatening condition and gaining sudden spiritual understanding and clarity, somehow I no longer felt the need to get definitive answers for all of life's questions. Due to the nature of my mind, I still immensely enjoy a good debate on these topics with my friends and even strangers at times as long as they do not take these matters too close to heart and are open to discussion. The limitless wisdom that exists in religion's vast ancient history and the current spiritual traditions could keep me learning for a lifetime and beyond. However, the burning need to understand and explain every aspect is no more. That which I am unable to explain rationally, comes to me on a different level, beyond words and reasoning, via direct experience with the higher power. In addition, comfort, peace and happiness are present whenever I reach out to that power through meditation.

Being human and living in a physical world, I am still not immune to disappointments and setbacks. I am always aware of the multiple "things to do," and some of them are, by their nature, frustrating and disappointing. Sometimes my efforts have succeeded, and other times, I faced multiple setbacks, of which I ultimately accepted and learned. (By the way, for each door that closed, another one always opened; and it provided opportunities that turned out to be far better than my original plans.) Life will always have ups and downs, successes and failures, accomplishments and disappointments. It is imperfect, and so am I.

I now have comfort, relief, personal knowledge and experience with the fact that when the physical world gets the better of me, or I start to lose focus, gaining it back is as easy as closing my eyes, taking a deep breath, and bringing me back to the source of it all. At that moment, I am once again "in the zone." The amazing thing about it is that the tools to do so are already in me and always have been. It was simply a matter of acknowledging and using them. The time that it takes to get "in the zone" can be as short as a moment. Within a blink of an eye, I can experience a new beginning, comfort, beauty, and happiness beyond anything that I have ever imagined. It has nothing to do with my physical possessions, status, or anything else in the outside world, for that matter. THE POWER IS WITHIN AND IS ALWAYS THERE. IT IS MY CHOICE TO ACKNOWLEDGE AND USE IT.

This is my story, my experience and my perspective. It has been shaped by my genetics, experiences, attitude, and many other factors too numerous to mention or even think about. YOUR STORY IS DIFFERENT BUT NO LESS REAL OR IMPORTANT. This is what has worked for me, and it is a miracle that I received, in part, thanks to what could have been both a physically and emotionally horrible experience (a diagnosis of cancer). For me, learning to connect with the higher power has helped me in ways that nothing else ever could. It led me to experience what Buddha would have likely called spiritual "enlightenment," and it saved my life. I don't know what the future holds for me, but I don't need to know either. I am comfortable with that. Every day that I wake up, I am more alive than I have ever been, and the joy and beauty of life is so powerful that I find it hard not to smile. I have no fear of physical death or, for that matter, any injury (physical, emotional, financial). I have no fear of life or regrets, only lessons from my mistakes so I can make better choices the next time. My heart is full of love and compassion, and it brings me even more pleasure to share with others.

As far as the subject of this book—in particular, weight loss and maintenance—it is close to my heart. I have always been aware of physical fitness and wellness, but one day, I discovered my future involvement in this area. It all started after watching a television program advertising a weight loss product. I do not, at this point, remember the name or the nature of the product itself, but it included the following: *before and after pictures; a spokesperson in a white coat claiming to be a weight loss expert; the claim that with the use of this product, there was no need to change one's diet, activity or lifestyle; and a guarantee to lose a lot of weight.* The phrases "magic bullet" and "fast and easy" were used without hesitation.

This became my trigger for focusing on further medical training in this field. The more I immersed myself in it, the clearer it became that wellness is my life's calling and something that I would actively pursue from that moment on. Thus, I set out to gain more expertise in the medical and scientific aspects of weight loss or "bariatrics" (Greek root "baro," as in weight). Bariatrics is the branch of medicine that deals with the comprehensive treatment of being overweight, including diet and nutrition, exercise, behavior modification, lifestyle changes, and medications when appropriate.

I took more medical courses, joined the American Society of Bariatric Physicians, and undertook a program to learn and to get board certification in Bariatrics. I subsequently passed the oral and written aspects of the board examination. Since then, I founded a medical weight loss practice called "Physician Weight Loss and Wellness Center." I also became a medical director for Tri-State Bariatrics, where I worked together with a surgical weight loss team providing a comprehensive, A-to-Z program for those trying to lose weight. The result has been a successful program with hundreds of patients and thousands of pounds lost in both the short and long term. While working with patients, I discovered one consistent factor behind successful weight control: empowering the individual to take ownership of their body, their progress and their life. This is what I call the "Power Principle." The idea of this book is to reach out to people who are trying to or are thinking of losing weight and acquaint them with the Power Principle.

Each person's life journey is unique and different from anyone else's and may involve, to varying degrees, the mind, body and spirit components, as well as different cultural beliefs, backgrounds and life experiences that shape and affect a person's thoughts, actions and perceptions. My sincere hope and ultimate purpose is to take the totality of my own life's experiences, knowledge, and skills to fulfill what I have realized is the most important purpose of my life. This is to help you achieve the "Power of You." In doing so, this book will:

- help you understand how to reach your goals and aspirations in weight loss and maintenance;
- give you the most accurate, applicable, up-to-date information and understanding;
- provide effective tools and ongoing motivation on your personal journey to weight control, including your current weight loss program and long-term weight maintenance.

Furthermore, I hope that the Power Principle, once realized and experienced, will also help you in all other aspects of your life in addition to weight control. THE ULTIMATE GOAL IS THAT THIS BOOK WILL BECOME YOUR STARTING POINT AND A GUIDE ON YOUR WAY TO REALIZING THE GREATEST TOOL THAT HAS EVER EXISTED, THE POWER OF YOU.

A line from the movie "Schindler's List" goes something like this: "To save (or help) one life, is to save (or help) the world." I certainly hope that I have accomplished that with this book and my practice.

Dr. Sergey Sorin

THE POWER PRINCIPLE

The body image issue and weight control have been a hot topic for centuries and, possibly, since the beginning of humanity. While the health aspects and focus on chronic disease prevention and control may appear to be a recent phenomenon, the benefits of a healthy lifestyle, proper diet and weight loss for those who are overweight have been well-known for a long time. In response to high consumer demand and interest, industrialists have developed an overwhelming number and types of "weight loss solutions" dating back to the 18th century and quite likely far before that. Even now, it appears that the new trends and diet alternatives are offering "The Magic Bullet," "New and Improved," "Natural" products. The plans and products include anything from fad diets, self-help programs, television competitions, cosmetic procedures, and even physician-based programs. The Internet, in fact, has thousands of books, articles, and plans claiming to have an answer to the weight loss. Meanwhile, the obesity rate in the United States is still at a record high and keeps climbing, so obviously, something is missing from the overall picture. That something is simple, very well known, based on common sense, and available at no cost whatsoever. The bottom line secret to effective weight loss and management, as well as lifestyle choices, is THE POWER PRINCIPLE.

Quite simply, only one thing can lead to effective and long-lasting changes that you desire, and it resides within you. WHEN YOU DECIDE TO MAKE A CHANGE IN YOUR LIFE AND COMMIT TO THAT CHANGE, THE COMBINATION OF DESIRE, KNOWLEDGE, AND SKILL (PRACTICE) WILL DETERMINE SUCCESS.

I often see commercials for weight loss products and services promising anything from "no exercise or diet changes required," "fast and easy," "the only thing you need to succeed," "guaranteed weight loss." All these ads and others of a similar nature have one thing in common. They place the focus of power on something external, "a magic bullet," such as a meal plan or a capsule, with the net effect of avoidance of personal responsibility and effort. Not surprisingly, the obesity and overweight epidemic is still here, and most people end up bouncing from one such "magic" program to another without losing weight in the long term and often even gaining weight. In the end, some will eventually conclude that it is impossible for them to succeed and stop trying altogether. HOWEVER, THE ONE THING THAT THEY NEED TO SUCCEED IS RIGHT THERE, EASILY WITHIN REACH AND ATTAINABLE. IT IS FREE, ALWAYS HAS BEEN, AND IT DOES NOT REQUIRE ANY OUTSIDE FACTORS.

The chapters that follow will serve as a guide to the most current information and principles, as well as interesting and perhaps not-so-well-known basics about weight control. This should act as your starting point on your weight loss journey, providing life-changing information to avoid the multiple pitfalls – yours, society's and marketers'. As you read on, you will learn to use the greatest tool that has ever existed – the Power of You. Based on my life experiences, as well as my experience as a bariatrician (weight loss specialist), once this power is cultivated, you will achieve both your short-term and long-term goals.

Part I
SPIRIT

CHAPTER 1

Life's Driving Force

One client, a pleasant man in his early 40s, has been significantly overweight since childhood and had tried multiple popular diet plans, including Weight Watchers, Jenny Craig, and the South Beach Diet. He even tried using doctor-prescribed weight loss medications, being evaluated for thyroid and other medical conditions possibly related to weight gain, and seeing a nutritionist. Despite all these attempts, nothing he tried lasted for more than a few weeks or had a significant long-term effect on his weight, which had been consistently climbing.

By the time he came to me for a weight loss consultation, he seemed to no longer believe in his ability to succeed. During our discussion, I discovered that there was very little I could teach him about nutrition, diet and exercise. Because of his experience, as well as being a highly intelligent man with a doctorate's degree, he could actually give me a lesson or two. So, instead of focusing on the details of *what* to do about his weight, I asked him to tell me more about *why* he was still struggling to lose weight despite his believing that he was unable to truly succeed.

Even though he was not a particularly religious individual, he did express a strong sense of obligation to his wife and children, and he was acutely aware that his weight made being a part of their lives more difficult. Furthermore, as the main provider for the family, he was afraid – rightfully so – that the weight would affect his health and the ability to continue taking care of his family. This was *the* turning point in our conversation. Now, instead of merely trying another "diet plan" with the anticipation of failure, he had a mission and a focus that was higher than a number on a scale.

We talked and agreed that this mission was going to be a lifelong process. There would not and could not be another dieting failure, only setbacks that could be overcome while on his path toward better health and goal of being there for those he cared about. He himself was no longer the focus of success or failure, so the pressure was off him. He no longer focused on how much he would lose but how much he wanted his family to gain by his enduring presence. His spirit came alive, for he was motivated by and wanted something greater than a physical manifestation.

Building on his prior weight loss experiences and already knowing what would and would not work for him, we put together a plan that included dietary, lifestyle, activity and exercise changes. He then began to see me on a regular basis. Even though he had days and even weeks at time of setbacks, he did stay with on a weight loss program for the first time in his life, and he felt confident in the progress he was making. Turned out, he did have the capacity to succeed; he just needed the proper motivation.

Having a lack of vision, connection to your higher power or a set of principles and priorities allows for the shifting of goals and waning of motivation. This deficiency is the typical situation with Yo-Yo dieters, whose pattern is about 4-6 weeks on point and then off again.

When we allow our current state of mind or outside circumstances to affect our attitude and actions, we are reacting versus acting. People who act do so with purpose and have a goal in mind. On the other hand, people who react fall prey to other people's whims and purposes. They either have no direction or seek direction. This lack of conviction affects every facet of their lives, including their weight and health management. Those who react to being overweight commit to diet and exercise for only a limited time. Those who take action about their weight have found a greater purpose for their lives and desire to lose weight to attain that end.

To gain spiritual direction needed to overcome obstacles, get and stay in touch on a regular basis with your higher power principles. For those who are religious or subscribe to a particular faith or spiritual practice, it is important to maintain prayer and contact with the higher power. For those who are spiritual, but not necessarily religious, the practice of meditation, which can serve the purpose of simply centering oneself or can become a part of the religious experience as one chooses, is a valuable exercise. Mediation enables people to abandon their preoccupation with the body and mind, instead awakening their consciousness of the spirit. Even if prayer or meditation has not been a part of your life and you feel that it will not work for you or cannot be beneficial in your circumstances, you can still realize your higher motivation or power source through other means.

For instance, Confucianism emphasizes self-cultivation and personal commitment to morality rather than abiding by explicit rules. Confucius, a Chinese philosopher and teacher born in 551 BC, had a profound effect on China's cultural and social aspects for more than 2,000 years until the Communist takeover in the 20th century. The basic premise of his teachings emphasized developing individual values and diminishing the ego. For example, the concept of "ren," or compassion for others, was central to the idea of showing more concern for others than oneself.

Either way, the purpose in connecting to the spiritual component is to seek and stay in touch with that which is higher and more permanent than the current, momentary self, which is a function of feelings, emotions, physical condition and life circumstances. The spirit is the guiding light, the permanent in the constantly shifting world and is the anchor that keeps us on the right track.

The body usually follows the mind. As far as the mind, it can be our greatest ally or our greatest enemy. It can set us up on the way to achieving greatness or can undermine our success, even if we are physically capable of achieving it. The good news is that we possess something much greater than the mind. That something is the spirit through which we connect to a higher power that gives us true purpose. Whether you are religious or not or subscribe to a particular way of life, most of us are driven by something. That something is greater than we are and is the reason we act as we do or try to accomplish a goal. If we retain focus on that higher purpose or power that drives us, then even when the mind starts heading in an unwanted direction, it can easily be brought back onto the right track.

Once you – whether religious, spiritual or value based – discover and/or establish that higher center, you must keep up the effort to maintain it and keep track of your relative position to it. As life's circumstances constantly change, losing track is "natural" and easy unless you are aware of and looking for it. As for prayer and meditation, my recommendation and personal practice is at least two times a day: in the beginning of the day and at its end.

Personal Worksheet for Discovering the Power of You

Getting in touch with the "Spirit":

Designate a quiet time when you can be alone and undisturbed for at least a few minutes. Clear your head, and take a few deep breaths. When the mind is as clear and still as possible, reflect on your life, and without trying to force it, let the feelings and thoughts pass through. Try to avoid analyzing, judging or reacting to them. Unlike passing emotions, which can be loud, intrusive, and overwhelming, the truly essential and important will present itself and will be a source of calm, comfort and support. Thus, the discovery of the "spirit" begins. It may take more than one session, but most people will find the practice to be quite enjoyable and relaxing, more of a reward than work.

Note: Those who are new to meditation and similar practices may find this difficult at first, but with more practice, they will find it very helpful. Even if as a result, one can only think of fitting into an old pair of jeans, for example, that in itself is an important insight.

Aligning the Spirit-Mind-Body axis:

Once you have an idea of what is truly important, it is then time to examine your current life situation and take stock of where you are and what you are doing now. Are your thoughts and actions in line with your higher motivation from the "spirit"?

In this regard, writing down and evaluating your daily activities may be a good practice. Those practices that are in line with the spirit's motivation should be continued, while those that are not should be re-evaluated and reconsidered.

Keeping up with change:

It's been said that the only thing constant is change. As life circumstances change, so does the need to re-evaluate and adjust accordingly. The good thing about being in touch with the "spirit" is that it can serve as a "lighthouse" to guide and direct even as emotional and physical factors are subject to flux.

Part II
MIND

CHAPTER 2

Intrapersonal Development: Getting on the Right Track

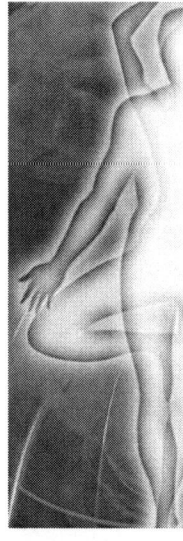

A very pleasant and cheerful woman came in for weight loss consultation. She described a long history of Yo-Yo type dieting effects with more weight re-gain after each diet attempt. When she came to the clinic, she was at her heaviest, but otherwise, the other aspects of her life seemed to be going well.

Initially, she responded well to a diet and exercise regimen and lost several pounds within a week, but she then regained the weight and came back to the office with "plan not working." Several modifications later and she had the same Yo-Yo effect.

During a follow-up visit with more thorough questioning, she shared her history of emotional/sexual and physical abuse in her younger years. Furthermore, I discovered that while maintaining an outward cheerful appearance, deep inside, she did not like herself, felt depressed and feel that life was not worth living. Being aware of the danger of being overweight on her health and well-being, she described her history of weight issues as "committing a slow suicide" even though she never actually took an "active" step to hurt herself.

With this painful realization accompanied by many tears, she was able to come to terms with the fact that all the years of Yo-Yo dieting had much to do with her own subconscious compromising her own efforts. At that point, my advice to her was to stop trying to lose weight and to first deal with the emotional trauma and its consequences on her life and mindset.

After some time, she did return to the program. This time, though, she had a new perspective, having also enlisted the help of a psychotherapist. For the first time in her life, she enjoyed a fair amount of weight loss and maintenance success.

The Power of You stems from and is ultimately based within each individual. As such, success starts from within, and it then becomes a physical reality. Most people who start on a weight loss program are extremely motivated at the start, but usually at about 6 to 8 weeks into the program, the motivation and the drive start to wane. The old habits then take over with a usual "Yo-Yo" weight loss and gain cycle. In my weight loss practice, I often see people who have successfully lost a certain amount of weight with various programs, but even after weight loss surgery, they regain the weight and sometimes more than their previous weight. The typical story is that "the diet didn't work," and "no matter what I do, I just can't succeed." Upon thorough questioning and a more detailed examination of the person's history, doctors learn that after the initial weight loss, the person went back to the same lifestyle (eating habits, inactivity, and other aspects) that led to the original weight gain. Rarely in these cases does the person incorporate lifestyle and dietary changes that they can maintain. While the possibility exists that the diet plan itself was not based on the right principles, or the person received a fair amount of misinformation; it is more likely that the diet did not fail, but rather the person gave up on the diet. This is often the case when one thinks of weight loss as a temporary solution without looking at it from a long-term maintenance perspective. With few exceptions, which we will discuss later in the medical conditions and medications sections, the obstacle to weight loss is not external, but lies within. This is where most of our efforts and energy must be focused.

Mental States that Affect Weight Loss and Control

Psychological Trauma: As in the example above, someone who has failed to deal with or has current or unresolved psychological issues will not likely do well with weight control. Part of it is due to the negative self-image or lack of belief in the self or capacity for achievement. In some cases, weight gain can even be a "shield" to avoid having to deal with the outside world or a subconscious effort to avoid attention. Also, it may serve as a means of self-punishment, especially if a person has feelings of guilt, regret or the like.

The problem is that weight gain and/or failure to lose weight cannot, by any means, resolve emotional or psychological issues. In fact, being overweight or having an undesirable external appearance can further negatively affect how we feel about our self-image and ourselves. The result is a downward spiral with seemingly no solution.

Unrealistic Expectations: Now this one is not entirely your fault. The self-centered society we live in is based on, and for that matter, relies on economically, instant gratification and being self-centered. This is how marketers have been able to manipulate and push their "new and improved" products and services.

Because our lives are so full of "things to do," traditional family ideals such as preparing home-cooked meals and dining with the family are being replaced by take-out and fast food. This hurried, instant lifestyle has affected all aspects of our daily lives, making multi-tasking a necessity for most people, including me. In this age, multi-tasking even makes sense in certain situations. For example, if a computer is having a problem starting up, simply waiting for it will not suffice. This delay is an indication that some other work can be done or started.

With having so many things to do and so little time, instant gratification is an integral part of our lives. If a microwave oven is not working, we often fail to even think of the stove as an option. This change in values can hurt us. Unlike a delay in a computer starting, weight loss is usually a long-term process. As I tell my clients, "This did not happen overnight and will not be resolved overnight, either."

While we may continue using the microwave and re-starting the computer or having it repaired if it's not working properly, we should take a different approach toward weight control. To gain long-term weight management, you must adopt a healthy lifestyle, or attitude, which means permanently changing your mind, not temporarily changing your behavior. A lifestyle is what it says, a style of life, and it should be established and maintained. Thus, your expectations of weight loss or control should not follow a six-week or less timeline.

Being overweight is something that emerged from the past, is now with you in the present and may likely affect your future. Therefore, this is one facet where the higher power should be constantly in unison with your mindset, and one aspect where instant gratification should have no role or priority.

Like our impatience, our self-centeredness, or ego, also affects our expectations. This is actually a significant aspect of the spiritual or higher power component as well. In 1920, Sigmund Freud widely introduced the term "ego" in the essay "Beyond the Pleasure Principle" and then later formalized and elaborated on it three years later in his "The Ego and Id." The concepts were later re-defined and extrapolated by Carl Jung, Alfred Adler, Otto Rank, Anna Freud, Margaret Mahler and others. Freud's original – and still highly controversial – description included three parts of the "psychic apparatus": id, ego, and super-ego.

Id was defined as the unorganized, unconscious part of the personality that is responsible for our basic drives, such as food, sex and aggressive impulses. It is further described as being ruled by the pleasure-pain principle and demands immediate satisfaction.

Ego was defined as the organized part of the personality structure, including defensive, perceptual, intellectual-cognitive, and executive functions. It mediates among the id, the super-ego and the external world with the task of finding a balance between primitive drives and reality while satisfying the id and the super-ego. Having to mediate between these three different factors, the ego is often in conflict and uses defense mechanisms to compensate for this constant struggle. Furthermore, it is said to be constantly monitored by the super-ego, which is at odds with the id.

Super-ego is described as the organized part of the personality structure that is mainly, but not fully, unconscious. It includes the individual's ego ideals, spiritual goals and the psychic agency commonly called "conscience," which criticizes and prohibits the ego/id drives fantasies, feelings and actions. Both ego and super-ego were said to be both in the conscious and unconscious realms.

The term ego has been used in multiple settings and with different meanings since. To Freud, ego is the part of the mind that contains the conscience, but other meanings of the term ego have emerged, including one's self-esteem, an inflated sense of self-worth and even one's self. In addition, the modern practice and study of psychiatry, psychology and behavior has many approaches to dealing with the ego. Some are aligned with the spiritual aspects while others are not. Furthermore, people have significant individual differences in terms of their beliefs, approaches and practices with regard to this topic.

The ego has been a subject of discussion and an area of focus of most spiritual and religious teachings, as well as at the forefront of the modern practice of psychology and psychiatry. Having completed a general review of the world religions including Judaism, Islam, Christianity, Hinduism, Taoism, and Buddhism, as well as non-religious spiritual movements, I have found that a common theme exists in them. The basic premise found universally is the presence of the divine or a higher than the individual self; elimination or at least subjugation of the ego; universal love; compassion for and service to others; living without fear, guilt and animosity. Similarly, many forms of prayer and meditation exist, but the universal purpose is to improve the quality of life, spiritual awareness, sense of purpose and direction, and understanding of being part of the greater force.

In our society, not only is the supremacy of the ego maintained but is strongly encouraged in our values. If it wasn't for this aim, perhaps the entire economic and social structure of the United States, as well as other countries, would be compromised. Consumerism relies largely on human dependence on external sources. However, uncontrolled ego can provide a sense of accomplishment and pleasure in addition to despair and discomfort. For instance, on one hand, we may be driven to work harder to be able to afford a house and certain lifestyle. On the other hand, once we do accomplish a goal, becoming unhappy or dissatisfied with what one has gained is quite possible, and thus we desire to get a bigger house and more things. We have no limit to our "wants." Likewise, the ego as described in this fashion is not the best or ultimate motivator for weight control either. We can never be too fit, too healthy, too attractive and so on. There will always be someone who is thinner, stronger and younger.

Understanding how the ego works and having a higher power can help overcome and deal with society's pressures and values. By being aware of your motivations, you can actively take steps to align your priorities and to map out strategies toward accomplishing that which is important. Following this path can also help with being pro-active (taking steps in the chosen direction) as opposed to being reactive (becoming a victim of circumstances and outside forces).

The First, Lasting Steps Toward Success

The first question you should ask yourself is: *"Why am I trying to lose weight?"* Is it because of health and well-being concerns? Is it to try to prevent and/or reverse medical problems? Is it to increase the fitness level? Or, is it for the purpose of "looking good for the summer?" While losing weight is certainly going to affect how you look, setting long-term goals and perspectives is much more likely to succeed, not only in the long term, but also in the short term. If you only consider the upcoming "bikini season" as your goal with no further long-term concerns, chances are that is exactly what will happen – you will look good for only that "season." Even if you do succeed in temporarily losing weight, after the summer, the efforts will stop and the weight will return for another cycle, likely with more gain than loss, and alas, the Yo-Yo dieting has started or is about to continue. On the other hand, keeping a long-term picture in mind will not only help you lose weight now, but it will keep you motivated after the weight loss to maintain it. Weight maintenance, by definition, requires not only having a weight loss plan, but also incorporating lifestyle changes and long-term dietary modifications that you can adopt for a lifetime.

In working from within, first you must take an honest look at yourself, your current habits and lifestyle that led to your current situation. During a routine consultation, most people can tell me exactly what got them in trouble. Usually it is inactivity, poor eating habits, including no portion control, too much fast food, eating out often, too many carbohydrates, eating late or eating while watching TV. For some, it is their hectic lifestyle and family situation. Many people mention stress and other forms of emotional eating. While each person has a unique situation and combination of factors, identifying the cause is usually easy.

Once you know what you need to work on, ask yourself, *"Am I worth it?"* That is, are you willing to rearrange your priorities to make yourself and your health a priority? If the answer is yes, then you can take the next step to identify and overcome the barriers that keep you from achieving your goals. You will have to make changes to your current lifestyle and habits, and this may be a difficult process. Most people are able to maintain their motivation for up to 6-8 weeks, but to break old habits and to incorporate new ones may take months, and to make them permanent, even up to a year. The following are some suggestions to help you move toward creating a healthy lifestyle:

Set the right goals: This is an important first step. Did you know that the amount of weight loss needed to improve your health may be much less than what you want to lose to look thinner? It's important to understand that your health can be greatly improved by a loss of 5 to 10% of your starting weight. That doesn't mean that you have to stop there, but this does mean that an initial goal of 5% to 10% of your starting weight is both realistic and valuable.

Most people who are trying to lose weight focus on one thing: weight loss. However, **focusing on dietary and exercise changes that will lead to permanent**

weight loss is much more productive. People who are successful at managing their weight set only two to three goals at a time. In order to be effective, goals should have three basic elements: specific, realistic and forgivable (less than perfect). As an example, "walking 30 minutes, three days each week" is specific, achievable and forgivable.

Set short-term continuous goals that move you ahead in making small steps to reach a distant point. At the same time, allowing continuous rewards (but not with food) for reaching those results keeps you motivated to make needed changes. Some examples of rewards may include material (e.g., movie, music, CD etc...) or an act of self-kindness (e.g., massage, personal time, etc...). For some people, keeping short-term goals with small rewards may be more effective than attempting long-term goals (requiring greater effort) with greater rewards.

Self-monitoring and consistency provide answers: Monitor your progress daily and keep physical activity, exercise and food diaries. This includes recording your caloric intake; quality of foods eaten; periods of lapses and the events surrounding them; amount of formal exercise, as well as activities of daily living (e.g., taking stairs rather than the elevator); and daily weight recording. In this way, you can monitor your actual behavior in comparison to your goals. Please keep in mind that one day's events may not make much of a difference, but a pattern of activity will. Consistency can identify both positive and negative patterns to make necessary adjustments or re-confirm your allegiance to following a fitness plan. In recording your daily weight, please be aware that variations may occur from day to day because of physiological factors, such as fluctuations in water retention and so forth. You should also be consistent in the use of the same scale and time of day for weigh-ins, such as in the morning after waking up or before dinner. Finally, creating graphs and charts of your weight, exercise pattern, and caloric intake may be helpful in giving a better indication of longer term progress and trends.

Know your triggers: If you have a known trigger for excessive or undesired eating, such as stress, watching TV, keeping treats on display or in proximity, then you should take steps to organize your environment in a way to protect yourself from temptation. For example, if you find that keeping snacks in a nearby place is a challenge, then make a conscious decision to limit the number of snacks in your surrounding area. Put them in places requiring effort to access.

Change the way you ingest food: After a meal, your body generally takes 15 or more minutes to perceive that it is full. Therefore, by eating slower and savoring the food, you will get to satiety with less caloric intake than you would ordinarily have. Eating more vegetables, soups, and drinking at least eight glasses of water can also help you feel fuller. Eating on smaller plates can make smaller portions look "bigger." Changing or setting an eating schedule so you don't skip meals and overeat later is also helpful, especially for those with work and home schedules that are anything but optimal. Schedule your needs into your day and make your health a priority.

Know your serving size vs. portion size: Pay attention to the amount of food you actually consume. The amount of food you are served or decide to eat is the "portion size," but the amount of food specified on the nutrition label is the "serving size." For example, one serving size may contain 100 calories, but if your portion size is 10 times that amount, then multiply the calorie level by 10. Different people have different caloric needs depending on their age, gender and lifestyle, so their portion size will vary slightly. The Food Pyramid provides general daily serving requirements, but a doctor or a nutritionist can provide more specific personal information.

Regular physical activity works for long-term goals: Exercising or engaging in some type of physical activity for 30 minutes a day at least five days a week will help you lose the weight and, more importantly, to keep it off. The benefits of regular physical activity include long-term physical and emotional health.

Prepare for the cycling nature of the problem: Weight control is a marathon, not a sprint. Even with successful weight loss, you may regain some of the weight at some point in your life. Do not worry. This simply means that you must return your attention to this issue again.

Most important of all, keep a long-term perspective and your true priorities in mind. You have decided that you are worth it and will make lifelong changes, not just temporary fixes. Most people who have tried previous diets have experienced a setback followed by a mind-frame of having "failed" or "can't do it." Others have gone through a phase best described as "cheating." The basic truth, however, is: *THERE IS NO SUCH THING AS A FAILURE!* In the spectrum of a lifetime, an isolated episode of "cheating," or a lapse, has almost no significance in setting a lifestyle pattern. You will not regain pounds during any one overeating episode or even after a few days of not monitoring yourself. As long as you are willing to get back on the plan and continue with it for most of the time, success will be yours. A temporary setback or problem only becomes a defeat if you let it and don't learn from it.

In my weight loss practice, I actually encourage people to go through these episodes every once in a while on purpose without feeling guilty or upset about them. How else can you learn about yourself and make improvements for the long term if you have no idea what to work on? Try to think of it from this perspective: fear, guilt, regret and shame are all mechanisms by which we can avoid taking responsibility for what happens to us. By removing these from your life or making an effort to do so, then when a lapse occurs, you have no other option but to acknowledge it and take the necessary action to deal with the situation at that time and preferably in all similar situations. Thus, a temporary weakness can now become a permanent strength and lifestyle change. As far as the term "cheating on my diet," you may want to think of the following analogy: If one cheats on a school exam, the goal is to improve one's grade or overall academic standing – morality and consequences aside, of course. If one cheats on his or her own diet, the effect only compromises the person's own success and effort. Essentially, it affects the individual, not anyone else. A dietary lapse is neither illegal by any means nor does it is affect others. So, is it really "cheating" in this sense?

The bottom line is: *Be good to yourself.* There will be times of difficulty and days (and even weeks) of lapses. Recognize these for what they are, opportunities to learn more about you and to make lifelong changes that improve the quality of your life and health. Also, this means no longer having to go through the Yo-Yo cycles of weight loss and regain, as well as the emotional and physical consequences of this. Give yourself the credit you deserve. Regardless of the amount of weight loss and progress, you are making your life better and being an active participant in writing your own life story and shaping your future.

Personal Worksheet for Intrapersonal Development

The first question you should ask yourself is:

Why am I trying to lose weight?
Think about it, and write down your top three to five reasons.

What is your anticipated time span?

Are you thinking in terms of a short-term goal or a long-term goal? While it is helpful to break down long-term goals into shorter segments (ex: 8 lbs weight lost in 1 month), having a life-long perspective is essential for staying on track and maintaining focus.

What are your strengths and weaknesses, and what can you realistically change now to start moving in the right direction?

Write down five or more observations about the above, and don't be too hard on yourself because you may be doing many things right already. Once you identify your weaknesses, choose three that you can start working on now. Keep in mind that it takes time, up to a year, to make habits permanent.

Am I worth it?

The important part once you know what it is you need to work on is to ask yourself if you are worth it. That is, are you willing to rearrange your priorities and to make you and your health a priority? I hope the answer is a clear yes! Otherwise, this may be a good time to go back and get in tune with your "higher power" through prayer and/or meditation.

Reflect on prior attempts to lose weight:

What worked well and why?
What did not work well and why?
Is there something you can learn from those events?

And please remember, there is no such thing as failure! Everything has a lesson.

CHAPTER 3

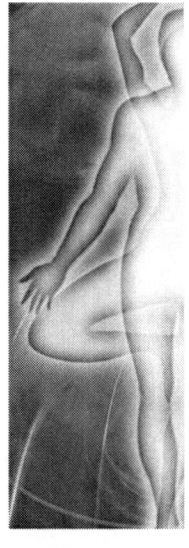

Interpersonal Development: Dealing with the Outside World

Once you have the drive and motivation to proceed with the weight loss program, you must also recognize the important effect that your environment has on success. I typically work with people who are doing all the right things within their capacity but who are dealing with an environment that is counterproductive to success. This may include the people in their lives, such as a spouse, parents, children, friends or co-workers who consciously or subconsciously compromise their efforts. This may also include an actual physical environment, such as a home pantry or desk full of junk food, a workplace where unhealthy eating is customary, and a neighborhood with doughnuts, pizza and sweets on every corner. The situation could involve a scheduling issue, such as shift work, overtime or excessive working, or a long commute.

Here's an example from my practice: One woman's husband initially encouraged her to lose weight, but he started becoming antagonistic once she started doing well. After sitting down with the both of them, I found out that he had become jealous of her as she was becoming more attractive to the opposite sex.

Realize that some outside factors, such as other people's attitudes, are easily dealt with while others will require more effort and adjustments. The bottom line is that **instead of spending lots of effort on "will power," which is important and does work well for some people, making changes to your environment or surroundings is often easier**. As far as the physical environment and arrangement, it varies for different people. However, the more changes you can make to align your home or work environment with your dietary plan, the less likely you will have a lapse or a "cheating episode." This may involve clearing out all the junk food and replacing it with high-quality food that is consistent with your diet. This may also mean placing the food further out of reach so that you will have to think twice before getting it as opposed to having it immediately available, which often leads to unplanned eating or snacking. For some, this process will be easy, but others will go through a "withdrawal" process. Just remember, **your current *lifestyle* is just what the word means: a way of life developed over a long period**. As such, noticing permanent results will take a long time as you adjust your environment and behavior.

Dealing with people, whether they are family, friends or co-workers, is another potential challenge. Some help you succeed in your goals, but others are standing in the way of your progress. As you may very well know, change is a difficult concept to accept and embrace even if it is for the better. Therefore, more often than not, you will face an initial resistance to your efforts. Part of this stems from a lack of understanding and information about the weight loss process and maintenance. Another aspect is that this process involves changing their perceptions and lifestyles, as well, if they are to agree.

In my clinical practice, I always advise and ask my clients to bring in the office their spouse, parents, children and anyone else who affects their lives. I then try to explain the process, reasons and the goals to everyone involved; and oftentimes, this is when the point becomes clear. If clients want to do this on their own, I recommend that they first gather all the information they are trying to communicate, set a time to talk, and then make sure that everyone understands. In terms of personal communication, some people may be easier to deal with than others. Also, different people have different styles of communication. In general, the best way to get your point across is being "assertive," which means being upfront and direct about your feelings and wishes, or "proactive," which means providing information before a situation occurs. This is different from being "passive," which means doing nothing to better or correct a situation, in that you do make your point. This is also different from being "aggressive," or confrontational, in that no blaming or arguing is necessarily involved. It is best to focus on statements such as "my needs are…," instead of "you are…" or "you do…" The word "you" causes people to become defensive, but "I" and "my" causes them to focus on you and not themselves. Another way to get people to be on your side is to recognize and sincerely appreciate what they have done or are doing that is positive. Dale Carnegie's books, including "How to Win Friends and Influence People," provide more advice on successfully dealing with other people.

In my experience, most people will be understanding of your needs and will become active participants and allies in your journey. Not surprisingly, in my own practice, often the whole family, not just the clients, ends up losing weight and becoming healthier. This is especially pertinent if you are not the one who typically cooks and buys food items.

Dealing with co-workers may be more difficult, as they may bring in foods that are bad for you and may not have your best interest in mind. Furthermore, some people may not feel comfortable discussing their weight concerns and lifestyle issues at work, so co-workers may be unaware of the dieting person's needs. In this case, minimizing the effects of the environment may be more difficult, but other ways still exist. For example, you may choose to bring your own food or not sit next to the snacks. You may also clear your desk of junk food and organize you personal space in a way that is conducive to your needs.

Lastly, **you may want to consider if your job, work hours, commuting distance, or personal situation is in line with your goals**. Some people and situations are easier to change or modify, but some seem more difficult. If you notice that something or someone is working against you, and you have the capacity to change it, then, by all means, do it. Just remember, you are worth it!

Here's an example from my practice: A client who for the last couple of years had a sedentary job and accumulated lots of pounds decided to switch career paths to something that involved more physical exertion. As a result, she was much happier and healthier in addition to losing weight.

Unfortunately, we cannot change some things, or they are harder to change. For example, if you are the main provider for the family, you may have a limited choice about commuting, work hours, or anything else, otherwise. Remember, you can always find some type of resourceful solution if you are determined. A long commute, irregular or long work hours, or a busy home routine does not necessarily mean poor food choices and timing. Knowing your goals and how you will get there, you can pre-plan meals for the day or week to stay with the plan as much as possible. Bringing a healthy food option with you during a commute or preparing a breakfast, lunch, dinner, and snacks consistent with the quality and quantity of your dietary plan will keep you on track. (Just please keep in mind that eating while talking on a cell phone and driving at the same time is still not a good idea in more ways than one.) Furthermore, that would eliminate the need for those foods that are bad for you, as well as allow you to time your food intake to a pattern that will work for you. Most of all, be patient with yourself, and give yourself credit for attempts, as well as accomplishments. Not every day will be great, but if you maintain an overall pattern of a healthy change, you will succeed.

Once again, remember that you are a priority and the reason for the changes, and you are worth it! Once again, there is no such thing as a failure. Each new day is a new beginning. **Do not hesitate to make your environment work for you, and do not become a victim of your environment.** You do have the power!

Personal Worksheet for Interpersonal Development

As you proceed with the diet, there may and likely will be days when the caloric intake and composition will exceed the above mentioned plan, or you will have the foods that you did not intend to have. Certain times you may feel frustrated or otherwise lose focus. Just remember that any one particular day or week is not nearly as important as the overall pattern of dietary intake in the long term.

What was the lapse?

Does it occur in a pattern? Are particular individuals, settings, etc.

involved?

What changes to your surroundings or environment can you make to help yourself stay with the plan?
List about three to five or more and how you will actually make it happen.

What challenges do you anticipate with the people in your life? Also, who can you count on to help you?
Make a list of those who affect you the most, and what you will do to address them.

Part III
BODY

CHAPTER 4

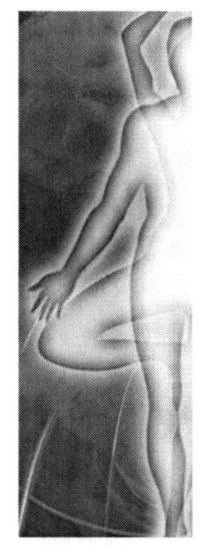

General Principles for Safe and Effective Dieting

With so much emphasis on being thin rather than necessarily being both healthy and thin, many popular weight loss methods range from risky to potentially dangerous. When choosing a diet plan or program, you should consider both health and maintenance, as well as weight loss. Factors to include are: appropriate calorie level, practicality, safety, maintainability, and most importantly, health.

To lose weight, you must intake less calories than your body needs or burn more calories than you intake. Typical caloric requirements for weight maintenance are: 2,300 to 2,900 calories/day for men; 1,900 to 2,200 calories/day for women. A rough formula for calculating the calories to maintain the weight is the following:

Male: 12 x weight (in lbs) x activity factor

Female: 11 x weight (in lbs) x activity factor

Activity factor is as follows:
Sedentary:	1.2
3 aerobic events per week:	1.3
5 aerobic events per week:	1.5
7 aerobic events per week:	1.6
Endurance athletic training:	1.7

"Weight in pounds" is applicable to the lean body weight more so than total weight. It can be deduced by first calculating the percent of body fat and then subtracting that amount from the total weight (see more about weight maintenance in Chapter 11).

Common Types of Diets

Balanced Caloric Deficit Diet: These diets require you taking in less calories than you expend, which is your "baseline calorie amount." This is the quantity of food (amount of calories) you would need to ingest to maintain your current weight, meaning you would neither gain nor lose weight. To determine your baseline calorie amount, try to maintain your current weight by tracking your diet and weight for at least two weeks. If a person is able to calculate or estimate his baseline calories required for weight maintenance, then he could conceivably decrease his calorie intake for the desired amount of weight loss. In general, a 500-calorie daily deficit will produce one pound per week weight loss because one pound of fat equals 3,500 calories. Thus, to lose two pounds per week, one would take their maintenance caloric needs and subtract 1,000 calories on a daily level. While in theory this is a viable alternative, determining the exact calories required may be difficult, and one may want to first experiment with different levels of intake and track the results of the weight loss. Usual goals with these diets are one to two pounds weight loss per week.

Low Calorie Diet (LCD): This diet involves keeping the caloric intake between 800 to 1,500 calories per day for overweight people. The most common is the 1,000 to 1,200 level, but some people will not lose weight until they go below 1,000 calories daily, typically 800-1,000. Likewise, some people who are physically active and have a larger frame or have more lean body mass will still lose weight when ingesting under 1,500 calories per day. Interestingly enough, a phenomenon occurs whereas those who are on a caloric restriction (example 1,000 calories) start to experience a plateau in weight loss after some success. In this case, increasing the caloric level by 100 to 200 calories per day may help to switch the body from an energy conserving (low metabolism) mode to energy expanding (calorie burning mode). Usual weight loss is about one to two pounds per week, but this may be less or more depending on other factors.

Very Low Calorie Diet (VLCD): This diet requires 400-800 calories per day for people with body mass index (BMI) over 32. (See Appendix C on how to calculate your BMI.) Weight loss can exceed three to five pounds per week and may be even greater for some individuals. **Physicians have to monitor these diet programs, and they are not recommended without medical supervision** (see section ahead on FAD and starvation diets). The reason for this is that providing balanced nutrient composition while ensuring healthy weight loss is difficult. One must also be careful to maintain a vitamin and other micronutrient balance. This can be accomplished by either using micronutrient-fortified products or taking multi-vitamin supplements. Most commercial A to Z products will do the job. Because getting proper nutrients is difficult to do with regular processed food, this diet often requires specialized meal programs, and may lead to blood chemistry and other abnormalities, thus, requiring strict medical supervision and monitoring.

The other aspect of the VLCD is that while the weight loss is more significant, it does not allow as much opportunity to develop changes and habits required for a healthy lifestyle. Therefore, one must be aware that the more rapid weight loss can be followed by weight regain, especially if a program does not incorporate lifestyle changes and education for long-term success, as well as a transition plan from the diet to maintenance plan.

Counting Calories vs. the Exchange System

The core of every reasonable weight loss program is being aware of the amount of food, or calories, you intake. Some programs are based on counting calories while others use the "exchange" or "modified exchange system" (e.g. American Dietetic Association exchanges, the Weight Watchers' point system, the DASH Eating Plan). An exchange system has a set number of servings from each food group. Foods are grouped together because they have similar nutritional values and/or calories. Each serving of a food has about the same amount of carbohydrate, protein, fat or calories as the other foods in the group. Thus, any food in the group can be "exchanged" or "traded" to maintain a certain calorie level. For example, you can trade a slice of bread for a ½ cup of cooked cereal (oatmeal) instead. Each of these foods equals one starch choice. For those who use the Internet, **http://www.MyPyramid.gov** is a helpful, free resource with a substantial amount of information, including the various food groups and exchanges, as well as other dietary recommendations.

Types of Diets to Avoid

Fad Diets: Every once in a while, a new diet emerges that claims to have a significant effect on weight loss. Upon closer examination, a pattern emerges that often includes the following: restricting a major macro-nutrient beyond what is reasonable, claims that "no exercise or lifestyle changes are necessary;" frequent use of the before and after pictures and testimonials; use of celebrities or other known public figures to increase the credibility effect; and some even have a statement such as "doctor approved" and may have an individual in a white coat presenting the information. An example of a fad diet is the "cabbage soup diet." The plan revolves around eating only cabbage soup in limited fashion. While cutting the calories and allowing a temporary weight-loss effect, the long-term effect often causes a deficiency in protein and essential fatty acids, as well as vitamins and minerals, which may produce health problems down the line and, more often than not, is followed by a rebound weight gain, often more than the prior weight.

Starvation diets or self-imposed fasts: These diets are quite common in people who want to lose weight quickly. They are often less than 800 calories per day and fall in the category of Very Low Calorie Diets (VLCD) except that the composition of the diet is often insufficient to maintain the basic body functions and lean body mass. The VLCD should be followed and monitored in a physician-based weight loss program for a number of reasons already stated. Maintaining the required essential amino acids and fatty acids, as well as vitamins and minerals, while severely restricting one's calorie intake is difficult. Maintaining an adequate protein amount to protect the lean body mass during the fast is also hard.

Often, while the weight loss can be significant during a starvation diet, the rebound weight gain almost always occurs. This happens for a number of reasons, including:

The person has a greater amount of lean body mass loss compared to fat loss, and this slows down the metabolism significantly. Thus, even if the individual goes back to a reasonable caloric level, maintaining the weight is difficult, and weight gain may occur on top of that.

Without lifestyle and activity changes, long-term weight loss is virtually impossible, and the old habits will take over once again (the ones that caused the problem in the first place).

With macronutrient, as well as vitamin and mineral deficiencies that result from starvation diets, the effect is to further decrease the metabolic rate.

With frequent rebounds and oftentimes more weight gain than the prior weight, many individuals become frustrated and conclude that they are unable to do anything about their weight. Once the person gives up, this self-perceived inability becomes a self-fulfilling prophecy, and a further Yo-Yo dieting effect or simply a lack of effort ensues.

In general, keeping the diet LEAN and GREEN, mostly consisting of lean proteins (8-16 oz. or exchanges), fruit (1-4 servings per day), vegetables (preferably non-starchy), as well as oils, will provide enough protein, complex starch, and essential fatty acids, fiber, vitamins, and minerals. As always, supplementing any calorie-restricted diet, or, for that matter, a typical high-calorie American diet, with a multi-vitamin, adequate fluids, a fish oil, or an omega-3 and omega-6 supplement is a good idea.

Personal Worksheet for Diet Plans

Do you recall a healthy diet plan that you were able to use successfully in the past for short and long-term success? Why did it work?

What did not work for you and why?

What resources and what kind of time can you devote to following such a plan?

CHAPTER 5

Recommended Adult Diet Plans

My personal recommendation for a starting diet is a high protein, low fat, low carbohydrate diet. For a male, a larger person or a very active person, it may be acceptable to have a caloric intake of 1,200-1,500 calories. For most women, those who are less active or those with a smaller bone structure, a diet of 800-1,200 calories will usually do the job. The following is my usual recommendation for a person who does not have a significant kidney problem or otherwise known inability to stay with a predominantly protein based diet.

High Protein Diets

With regard to fluids, stay away from high calorie soft drinks, fruit juices, and alcohol (7 cal/gm, as well as predisposition to excessive caloric intake). Recommended fluids are water (six to eight glasses per day is recommended or 64 oz. per day) and non-caloric beverages, such as Crystal Light and diet drinks.

Vegetables should be mostly green but may include starchy vegetables occasionally. An exchange is ½ cup cooked or 1 cup raw vegetable, which contains 25 calories and includes 5 grams of carbohydrates and 2 grams of protein. These tend to be high in fiber, vitamins and minerals, as well as low in calories (low caloric density). For this reason, vegetables should be a main staple along with protein-based products (see below). If in doubt, do not be overly concerned with how much non-starchy vegetables you intake. The caloric amount is insignificant, and they do tend to have a filling effect on the stomach in addition to the inherent high quality of the micro-nutrients (vitamins and minerals).

The way in which the vegetables are prepared is also important. The best way to preserve the vitamin and mineral composition is to steam the vegetables or have them raw when possible. Frying not only affects the quality of micronutrients but also adds lots of extra calories from fat. Using a one-calorie spray to prepare vegetables is highly recommended as long as the number of sprays is kept in control.

Here's an example from my practice: While the vegetables themselves are usually not the problem, you should keep track of the dressings used and how much. One client used so much dressing with vegetables that the calories from the dressing were more than from the rest of the meal.

Vegetables such as beans, rice, peas, corn, potatoes, carrots, and squash are categorized as starches, or complex carbohydrates, and contain approximately 15 grams of carbohydrates, 3 grams of protein and 0-1 grams of fat. The caloric amount in a serving (typically 1/2 to 1/3 of a cup) is 80 calories. Complex carbohydrates have three or more sugar molecules and are known as "good" carbs, and simple carbohydrates have one or two sugar molecules and are often called "bad" carbs. Unlike simple carbs, the body has to work hard to breakdown and absorb complex carbohydrates, so they can supply a steady source of energy without immediately being stored as fat. Because complex carbs have a more favorable glycemic index, they are preferable to an equivalent amount of simple carbohydrates, such as white bread and table sugar. Nonetheless, this category, whether a simple or complex carbohydrate, tends to have high caloric amounts and should be limited while on a low-calorie diet.

Fruits are a source of carbohydrates at 15 grams and about 60 calories per serving. Although carbohydrates in this category are of the simple type, they provide a good amount of fiber, vitamins and minerals and have a low glycemic index. Even with diabetes or insulin resistance syndrome, these are good as a snack, and a much better alternative to other simple carbohydrates used as ingredients in sweets. While on an 800-1,200 calorie diet, up to four or five servings are acceptable, or up to 240 calories per day. However, having that amount every day is unnecessary, but fruit does serve as a good way to enhance the taste of other foods or when used as a dessert.

Proteins are the staple of a low calorie diet, and they come mainly in both animal (meat, fish) and plant (nuts, beans, seeds) sources. They are essential for maintenance of lean body mass and great for appetite control. While taking into account the above-mentioned vegetable and fruit intake, the minimum daily requirement to maintain an 800-calorie diet is about 400 calories of protein. In terms of having low fat, lean protein sources, try baking chicken and certain types of fish. This can provide about 8 ounces or 100 grams of protein. If you don't have a small scale to weigh the meat in ounces, you could estimate that a 3-ounce portion of meat is about the size of a deck of cards or the palm of a hand. For fish, this is about the size of a checkbook. A 1,000-calorie diet requires about 600 calories of protein, or 12 ounces of very lean to lean meats/fish or an equivalent, corresponding to about 150 grams of protein. For a 1,200-calorie diet, you should intake 800 calories of protein with up to 16 ounces of a very lean to lean protein source, corresponding to 200 grams of protein.

When taking the amount of protein into consideration, you should understand that meats or fish vary in their calorie count based on their fat composition. As mentioned above, in terms of meat or meat equivalents very lean sources provide about 35 calories per ounce, lean 55, medium fat 75, and high fat 100. Thus, the protein source will significantly influence the amount of fat and calorie intake and should be adjusted appropriately based on your diet plan. (See Appendix G for specific examples of high protein, low carbohydrate, low fat diets at each caloric level.)

Balanced, Low Calorie Diets

Balanced, low calorie diets incorporate all the major food groups and can serve as an alternative to a high protein, low fat, low carbohydrate diet for those who either cannot let go of the carbohydrates, dairy and fats, as well as in cases where protein intake must be watched closely, such as in certain kidney diseases.

Low calorie balanced diets are in the range of 800 to 1,500 calories daily. Adult maintenance diets based on balanced diets are usually in the caloric range exceeding the 1,500 calorie level, up to 3,200 calories. (See the maintenance chapter for more information.) The use of balanced diets do not extend below the 800 calorie level, as this falls in the category of Very Low Calorie Diet (VLCD) and should be used only in a physician-monitored program. Otherwise, it may fall in the category of fad or starvation diet with potential harm to the body, as well as a tendency to regain an even greater amount of weight afterward. (See Appendix H for more information on specific balanced diet plans for different caloric levels. Included are guidelines for the 800-1,500 calorie level balanced diets.)

Personal Worksheet for Adopting a Diet Plan

Not all diets will work for all people. Use your own progress and experience to modify and adjust the caloric level and dietary composition to what you can maintain to achieve success. **In the end, the diet has to work for you, not you work for the diet!**

What foods group(s) would you struggle with minimizing or restricting?

Which are you more willing to do:

Change what I eat

Change the amount I eat

What, if any, health concerns would prevent you from using a high protein, low fat, low carb diet?

What, if any, health concerns would prevent you from using a balanced low calorie diet?

Based on your answers to these questions, you should be able to determine which of the two recommended diets* would work best for you.

*A physician or nutritionist consultation is recommended when deciding on the type of diet to pursue, especially if any health questions are involved.

CHAPTER 6

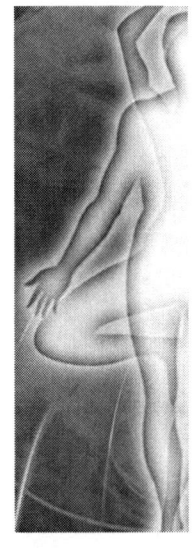

Weight Loss for Children and Adolescents

In 1999, 13 percent of children aged 6 to 11 years and 14 percent of adolescents aged 12 to 19 years in the United States were overweight. These numbers have nearly tripled for adolescents in the past two decades, according to a 2007 U.S. Surgeon General report. Overweight adolescents have a 70 percent chance of becoming overweight or obese adults. The possibility increases to 80 percent if one or more parents is overweight or obese, according to the same report. With children and adolescents, the principles of weight control are, in some ways, similar to adults, but there are also significant differences.

Here's an example from my practice: I saw an 8-year-old girl who was sent from school with a letter to see a doctor for her obesity. She saw the letter and was extremely upset at the recommendation. I explained to her and her family that, by definition, she cannot be labeled "obese" (see discussion below) as a child, but that she was "overweight" and at risk for obesity in years to come. After my explanation, they were able to accept and initiate a plan to address the problem. Immediately after the visit, she started with the activity part of the program by running a lap around the building.

In terms of similarities with adults, most children who are overweight have a contributing component of the following: genetic and familial patterns (tendency to be overweight when other members of the family are also overweight); the environment, especially in terms of dietary intake; activity (or inactivity) level; and the financial and social situation (in terms of being able to afford better quality food or safe housing). One way to look at the interaction of genetics and the environment is a gun-and-trigger analogy. Having genetic predisposition to being overweight is like having a loaded gun at the onset. The environment and lifestyle then act as a trigger in terms of weight gain.

Other factors that are similar to adults include the effect of dietary choices, activity level, and the fact that overweight children and adolescents are also subject to premature development of weight-related medical problems and complications, including diabetes, high blood pressure, joint problems and depression, to name a few. Dietary factors most often associated with childhood and adolescent weight gain are high fat and simple carbohydrate (sugar) diets; poor snacking and meal patterns; frequent visits to fast food establishments; and excessive amounts of soft drinks and juice. Activity patterns contributing to weight gain include a sedentary lifestyle; increased television, video games and computer-based activities (more than 1-2 hrs/day); and extrinsic obstacles to activity, such as unsafe neighborhoods and parental time restraint.

As with adults, effective treatment is also multifaceted, including dietary, lifestyle and activity changes. Starting at 12 years old, adolescents may also take certain medications, (see below for more details) including Orlistat (fat absorption blocker) at the age of 12 years old, and Meridia (appetite suppressant) starting at 16 years old. At 16, they may also have a surgical procedure depending on the surgeon's comfort level and approval, as well as other factors.

While overweight adults and children may share similar dietary patterns and treatment options, they also have significant differences. For instance, children must use a Body Mass Index adjusted for age (BMI-for-age) graphs as opposed to simply using a BMI (Body Mass Index) to measure their height to weight status. (See Appendix C for adults and D for children.) Some healthcare providers still may not be aware of this fact. For example, a 5-year-old may have a BMI of 22 (considered normal for an adult), but this child is significantly overweight using the BMI-for-age chart.

Unlike with adults who have four main categories (*underweight, normal weight, overweight* and *obese*) to describe their weight, children have an additional category (*at-risk for overweight*). This category is between normal weight and overweight, and it needs to be addressed before the problem intensifies. Also, the official term "obesity" does not apply to children, and instead, falls within the category of "overweight." The reason behind this is likely two-fold: to prevent emotional trauma associated with being labeled obese, and also given the ability of children to lose weight easier than adults due to rapid growth and a generally faster metabolic rate.

When it comes to children and weight, the family dynamics and parents' weight status is extremely important. Up to the age of 6 or so, the child's weight is mostly based on their family factors. Once the child gets older, parents and caretakers are less to blame, as older children start making more independent decisions and parental control begins to wane. However, even then, caretaker influence is extremely important in terms of role model behavior, meal preparation, and the environment and lifestyle within the household. Once parents or caretakers start working on their own health and lifestyle, children tend to follow as well. We commonly observe overweight children in the setting of overweight families rather than with families in which health and wellness is a priority.

All this being said, having an overweight child is not always a parent's or family's fault. Whether we like it or not, children (especially once they get older) have their own minds and make their own choices.

Treatment options also vary depending on the combination of age and weight status, or whether a child is at risk for overweight or already overweight. Definitions of overweight and at risk for overweight are as follows:

At risk of overweight: BMI-for-age between 85-95% for ages 2-20.

Overweight: BMI-for-age at or above 95% for ages 2-20

For children up to 2 years of age, physicians consider children's growth patterns, as well as their age, to determine whether their weight is healthy. Thus, you can use the weight for length and weight for stature charts often used in the pediatrician's office.

Goals of dietary interventions in children are as follows:

0-2 years old: monitor the growth curves

2-7 years old: with BMI-for-age at 85-95% (at risk for overweight), the recommended course of treatment is weight maintenance by modifying the diet and increasing activity. (There is a 5 lb weight loss equivalent with every inch of growth while maintaining weight.) With BMI-for-age greater than 95% (overweight) without medical complications (i.e. hypertension), the recommended course of treatment is weight maintenance, whereas with complications, weight loss is recommended.

7 years old or older: with BMI-for-age 85-95% (at risk for overweight) without complications, the recommendation is weight maintenance; whereas with complications, weight loss is recommended. When BMI-for-age is greater than 95% (overweight), the recommendation is weight loss.

In general, the following dietary interventions apply to children as they do with adults: a low fat, low glycemic index, high fiber diet; proper portion control; label reading; and non-food rewards for weight loss. For those children and adolescents who qualify for weight loss according to the BMI-for-age, see Appendix J for pediatric weight loss dietary guidelines. These pages can also serve as a tool for planning daily meals. Similar to adults, the use of a food diary is another useful tool. For those recommended to maintain their weight, see Appendix K.

Increasing activity is beneficial for both adults and children. In my experience as a bariatric physician with children, the use of a pedometer, which counts steps, significantly adds a dimension of fun and helps with the activity factor. For a balanced pediatric program of weight loss, a daily activity goal should be 10,000 steps (pedometer). Another recommendation is more than one hour of continuous, moderate activity regularly throughout the week.

Doctors and other healthcare professionals can provide a thorough assessment to determine the cause and treatment of your child or adolescent's weight issue. However, keep in mind that this topic is still not well known or being addressed adequately – even within the healthcare community. Proper medical evaluation of the overweight child is critical and should include testing for predisposing medical conditions, such as thyroid, as well as for conditions resulting from being overweight. This is important and relevant because childhood weight issues are very likely to continue into adulthood. Many of tomorrow's obese and overweight adults are today's children who are either overweight or at risk for being overweight. Furthermore, in terms of medical complications, children with weight-related issues are at risk for the same health care complications, including early onset diabetes or insulin resistance, high blood pressure, cholesterol, etc.

They also risk emotional problems, including depression, peer pressure and other significant factors.

Getting an early start and focusing on both health and weight is probably the best thing you can do for your child in terms of his or her health. Last, but not least, as the child gets older and gains more self-insight, the mind-body-spirit paradigm and self-determination become more important. The younger child is at an ideal stage to get on the right track to weight control and wellness. The earlier the process starts, the better the outcome, but it is never too late to start.

If your child does fall into the category of overweight, make sure to have a discussion with your child's health care provider regarding not only the need to address the weight issue, but also blood pressure, cholesterol, diabetes, and other weight-related complications. Being a child or adolescent does not protect or keep you from the complications of overweight or obesity. Childhood weight-related issues are still, unfortunately, not well known or addressed even within the healthcare community. Get to know your local resources and options.

Personal Worksheet for Parents of Overweight Children and Adolescents

Does anything in your or your family's medical history or genes indicate a potential weight issue with your child?

What kinds of food (fast food, balanced cooked meal, quick prepackaged meals) do you prepare or give your child on a normal basis?

Do you restrict your child's intake and amount of certain foods, or is your child basically allowed to eat what or how much he/she wants? If you do have restrictions, what kinds or amount of food?

As parents or caretakers, what are your own personal diet, nutrition, lifestyle and activity patterns? Are those the patterns you wish to instill in the child, and if not, what can you do to move in the right direction?

Do you expect your child to finish everything on his or her plate? Does the child typically get seconds or desserts?

How much time does your child spend daily on exercise or physical activity? If none, why?

What does your child feel about his or her weight?
(Remember, that a child is a person with his/her own mind, priorities and certain independent actions. If weight control is unimportant to children, chances are they will not respond to outside interventions. This is especially true for an older child or an adolescent.)

CHAPTER 7

Activity and Exercise

So where do physical activity and exercise enter the equation for weight loss? We all know that exercise is an important aspect of a healthy lifestyle, but many misunderstandings and misconceptions exist about the role and effects of physical activity with regard to weight management. Here are some basic facts:

Exercise and physical activity act as an independent factor in improving health and preventing health-related problems regardless of the effect on weight. Thus, even if weight loss is not desired or occurring, people still do well for themselves by increasing their activity level and initiating an exercise program. **Note: In the presence or possibility of health issues, I strongly advise consulting a physician for medical clearance prior to starting an exercise program or increasing one's activity level. This especially applies to people with known heart, lung, joint and bone problems, as well as those who experience chest pain, shortness of breath, significant pain, dizziness or any other problems during activity. A medical consultation is then highly advised as soon as possible.**

It is possible to be physically active and exercise and still be overweight or have a difficult time losing weight. Reason being, weight loss is still pretty much a function of calorie balance; if you intake more calories than you expend or burn, you will gain weight. The opposite is true for weight loss. Thus, if you consume fewer calories than you expend, you will lose weight. From my practice, I have learned that a strenuous workout that burns 400 calories is no match for a piece of cheesecake (easily exceeding 400 calories per small serving) that follows it.

A 30-minute exercise session, while great for cardiovascular conditioning and burning some calories, by itself, does not burn as many calories as being active throughout the day. In an average active person who tries to incorporate three to four exercise sessions per week, the caloric expenditure of one workout is only about a third of the total energy expenditure for the day. Thus, if a person leads a relatively sedentary lifestyle, other than the three to four workouts per week, the overall calorie burning is quite limited.

Being physically active during the day (ex: physically demanding job with lots of walking, lifting and other activity) is a great way to burn calories during the day, but in itself does not always provide the benefit of formal exercise in terms of cardiovascular conditioning or improving strength and endurance. Thus, even if a person is physically active, he or she should participate in a formal exercise program as long as no limitations or medical reasons occur for not exercising.

Monitoring the activity level and being aware of it cannot be emphasized strongly enough because most people tend to underestimate their caloric intake and overestimate their activity and exercise. To begin with, I recommend purchasing a pedometer, a device that measures the number of steps taken. The goal is to reach 10,000 or more steps per day. If one can go above this number to 15,000 or more, the energy expenditure and the effect on weight loss is much more pronounced, but 10,000 steps is a great level.

For people starting a weight loss program, they should first obtain the baseline or normal number of steps. While wearing a pedometer, just do what you normally do while awake during the day. Write down the daily number of steps and see what the average is for the week. (See Appendix E for a sample pedometer diary.) You may be surprised to see what that number is. Some people discover that they only generate under 1,000, and in some cases, less than a hundred steps per day. Others may already be at or above 10,000. Either way, the goal is to be aware of where you are and to try to improve on this. One way to do so is the following: Take the average number of steps for the week and multiply it by 1.2 (or an increase of 20 percent above the prior level). Try to stay consistently at or above this number (example: if your baseline is 1,000 steps a day for the first week, multiply 1,000 by 1.2. The number then becomes 1,200 steps, and this is the number to try to maintain for the next week. Increasing by 20 percent each week or every few weeks will get most people to their goal faster than they expected. Sometimes a problem such as arthritis, a heel spur, a sports injury or another medical concern may come along and cause significant discomfort. In this case, the best option is to stop and seek medical care to resolve those problems prior to proceeding.

As always, personal safety always comes first. Some people will start with a higher baseline number and will get to 10,000 steps or above in no time. That is great. However, others may begin with a low baseline. In my practice, some discover that their pedometer average is less than 100 steps a day, an extremely sedentary lifestyle indeed. In this case, the same principle still applies. Start from your baseline and increase by 20 percent as much as possible on a weekly basis. If you think about it, going from 100 to 1,000 steps per day may seem a long way from a 10,000 goal, but at the same time, this is a 10 times increase in the activity level, which is not a bad accomplishment.

The best way to use a pedometer is for what it is designed to be, a tool to raise your awareness of your daily activity. It is a tool – nothing but a tool. My recommendation on the maximal use of a pedometer is the following: Once you know your baseline and have established a certain goal, check your pedometer often or at least once during the day. If, for example, you are aiming for a 10,000 step average this week, and by mid-day you have only accumulated 2,000 steps, then you know it is time to find ways to increase your activity level. Conversely, the least productive use of a pedometer is not to use it at all.

A note on pedometers: Pedometers come in many shapes, sizes and functions. Some only count steps and others calculate your distance and calories along with multiple other functions. As far as pricing, they tend to vary from giveaway models at under $5 to over $40 to $50. In general, the more functions it provides, the more expensive it will be. It is important to understand a few things. Other than steps, a pedometer (with a few exceptions) is not designed to accurately measure anything else. So, my recommendation is to get the most basic model and focus on the 10,000-step goal. Choosing a model with more functions is a personal decision and may help with motivation, but will likely cost more. With regard to cost, the very inexpensive models (under $10 or those that are giveaways) are usually not of the greatest quality. They tend to break easily or significantly over-count or under-count the number of steps, thus defeating the very purpose of having a pedometer. If you have one in your possession and want to see if it works, then try walking a certain number of steps (example 100), and then see what the pedometer records. If it is close to 100, then you may consider using it, but check it periodically for accuracy. If it is very inconsistent, it is best to invest in a replacement. Most reliable pedometers are in the $20 range. The Digiwalker is the gold standard for use in research studies in addition to its proven reliability in my own experience. The basic model S200 starts in low $20's and only counts steps. Other brands of pedometers may also prove reliable, but whatever brand you choose, make sure to test it prior to use. As always, the choice is there to purchase a much more expensive model, usually with more functions, but again, with few exceptions, those functions are not as helpful as the number of steps.

The best combination is to undertake a formal exercise regimen 3-4 days per week that includes an aerobic activity, resistance training, and stretching components for 30 or more minutes per day in addition to leading or undertaking a more active daily lifestyle. Walking is a great way to get started with aerobic activity (try to increase the pace for at least 5 to 10 minutes of the walk). For beginners, walking for 5 to 10 minutes a day is a great start, and most people will increase the time, distance and pace as their cardiovascular level and muscle tone increases. Remember, a 10-minute workout is still better than nothing at all.

The best evidence for physical activity and exercise in the weight loss process is for its role in maintaining weight loss and preventing weight gain. Physical activity also plays a crucial role during times when the effect of a diet on the weight starts to reach a plateau despite maintaining the same caloric level. By increasing the activity level, one does increase the metabolic rate and calorie burning.

The three types of exercise include aerobic (walking, running, etc...); resistance (weights, machines, etc...) and stretching.

Aerobic is the most important type of physical activity for weight loss. It results in an improved cardiovascular status, calorie burning and muscle tone.

Several methods exist to see if you are at the right level of activity. Primarily, see how you feel during the activity. If you feel you can do more, it is a good indication that you can. On the other hand, if you are out of breath or can't talk during the activity, chances are you are at or above your maximum recommended heart rate and need to slow down. Another way is by monitoring the heart rate itself. There is a number of heart rate monitors and sports watches out there that will measure your heart rate. The formula for Maximal Heart Rate (MHR) in an otherwise healthy person is generally:

205 − (age / 2)

For a 20-year-old, it would be: 205 − (20 / 2) = 195

For an 80-year-old, it would be: 205 − (80 / 2) = 165

Unless you are in the middle of a strenuous workout routine or training for a competitive event, it is best not to exceed the maximal heart rate. In general, for an easy or prolonged workout, try to stay in the area of 65 to 75 percent of MHR. For a more challenging workout, try to be in 85 to 95 percent of MHR. Lastly, for an elite athlete or for someone in a hard training program, one can go up to 95 to 100 percent of MHR.

Resistance is an integral part of the workout as well. The benefits include muscle conditioning and building but may also have an aerobic component if done in rapid succession, or a circuit training workout program. In general, in order to benefit from resistance training, one needs to break down the muscle tissue, which then reforms itself (thus increasing mass and tone). With heavier resistance and fewer repetitions, one tends to increase muscle mass, while lesser resistance and more repetitions will likely improve the muscle tone without as much of an effect on muscle building. With regard to burning calories and metabolism, the more skeletal muscle one has, the higher the metabolic rate. In terms of timing, it may be beneficial to alternate body parts so that you do not work the same muscle group several days in a row. For example, do not do heavy bench presses several days in a row, allowing the body to recover and the muscle tissue to rebuild after being broken down during exercise.

Stretching is recommended with both aerobic and resistance activities to prevent injuries, improve joint flexibility and function, and obtain a greater range of motion. In the past, it has been recommended to stretch prior to the workout: but evidence is now pointing to stretching after the activity as the greatest benefit. In any case, stretching both prior to and following activity is not a bad idea.

Overall, for the purpose of weight loss and basic muscle conditioning, it is recommended to maintain a ratio of 75 percent aerobic activity to 25 percent resistance-based activity. In other words, for maximum weight loss, make sure to spend more time with calorie burning aerobic activity.

One way to get started with an exercise program is by joining a gym or hiring a personal trainer. You should get medical clearance for the program you would like to initiate, especially if you have any potential medical concerns.

You may also choose to begin a regimen at home by investing in your own equipment, i.e. a treadmill, exercise bike, gym equipment, tapes or DVD's, or any other equipment. *The bottom line is the program you choose to undertake should be reasonable to your lifestyle.* For example, it would be hard to start a swimming program if you don't regularly have access to a swimming pool, or the nearest one available is more than an hour away. Walking or running may be a more logical alternative. *The program should be enjoyable.* For example, it may not make sense to start running if you do not enjoy it, but you may enjoy swimming in your own swimming pool or at a nearby community center. *The program should be physical-*

ly possible. In other words, you may want to address the heel spurs that cause you pain while walking prior to starting a running program, or you may consider a stationary bike instead. Finally, the regimen should be something you can see yourself doing now and in the future. Some people stay with one routine once they get started, and others vary their exercise patterns, i.e. running on a treadmill during winter, and playing tennis outside when the weather gets warmer. Whatever it is you do, make a commitment and stay active as much as possible. On the other hand, there are also times to take it easy. If, for example, you discover that you are having chest pains on exertion or worsening shortness of breath with the same or even a lower level of activity, it is a good time to see your physician and get this checked. Likewise, if you get sick or develop any other problem along the way, it is best to stop and re-evaluate whether it is a good time to continue exercising. The last thing you want is to get hurt. This being said, without significant contraindications or physical problems, increasing your physical activity and starting a formal exercise program one of the best things you can do for your health!

Personal Worksheet for Exercise and Activity

What type of activities have you enjoyed in the past or do you enjoy now?

What types of activities can you think of that are possible, enjoyable, and sustainable? List 3-5 reasonable suggestions and the timeline for implementing them.

Can you think of any limitations or problems with exercise or activity and what can be done to overcome them?

Once you obtain a pedometer, get an average daily baseline number of steps over the course of the week. How close are you to achieving 10,000 steps a day or more? Decide on a plan to move towards your goal. (Can you increase the number by at least 20 percent every week or every few weeks?)

How can you change your daily routine or environment to automatically increase the number of steps and activity level? List 3-5 reasonable suggestions and the timeline for implementing them.

CHAPTER 8

Medical History and Weight Gain

As we have seen above, the problem of obesity and being overweight has far-reaching implications in terms of health, beyond simply one's appearance or reflection in a mirror. In fact, many medical conditions are closely related to and/or are at least in part caused by excess weight. These include diabetes mellitus (diabetes); high blood pressure, cholesterol, arthritis, certain forms of cancers, gallbladder disease, gynecologic and fertility disorders, and depression, among others.

Side effects of medications prescribed for some of the most common conditions can contribute directly to weight gain and/or difficulty losing weight. Some medical conditions can, in turn, have an effect on the weight loss process, making it more difficult to lose weight or resulting in weight gain, including but not limited to: polycystic ovarian syndrome, low thyroid function, diabetes, and certain endocrine (metabolic) and genetic conditions. Common endocrine associations that have a direct effect on the weight include the following: insulinoma (tumor of the pancreas), hypothyroidism, Cushing's syndrome, prolactinoma, polycystic ovarian disease, insulin resistance (previously known as Syndrome X), and type 2 diabetes (non-insulin dependent diabetes mellitus).

While the best way to go about addressing these concerns is to speak with your healthcare provider, below is some basic information on the most common medical conditions that affect weight loss and maintenance:

Insulinoma: This condition is a rare pancreatic endocrine tumor that is found more often in women (60 percent). The most common symptoms include confusion, forgetfulness, personality changes and unusual behavior, lightheadedness or dizziness, weight gain, sweats, tremors, fast heart rate, weakness, fatigue and blurred vision. As excess insulin production by the tumor leads to low blood sugar level (hypoglycemia), symptoms are usually relieved with eating. It is easily missed or will rarely be detected with only a physical checkup. In order to properly diagnose this condition, your healthcare provider must perform blood tests to detect glucose and insulin levels while symptoms are occurring. At the time of symptom occurrence, a positive diagnosis consists of the following: glucose level of less than 45 mg/dl; insulin level greater than 5 micro international units/ml; negative sulfonylurea screen (medication for diabetes); and negative insulin antibodies. If a person has no hypoglycemia (low sugar) during the required 72-hour fast, most likely this condition will be excluded.

Hypothyroidism: The thyroid hormone functions to regulate the metabolic rate, maintain body temperature, allow for energy production, and is essential for the functioning of all cells. The body has developed a very precise and complicated control mechanism in order to produce the right amount of this hormone. One analogy would be to think of TRH (from the hypothalamus gland in the brain) as the owner of a factory who sends a message to a middle manager (TSH from the pituitary gland) to increase production of units of thyroid hormone. The middle manager (TSH) then, in turn, sends a message to the factory workers to produce more units of T4 and T3 (thyroid hormones). T4 and T3 then go to work on the different body organs and cells to produce the thyroid effects. When too much thyroid hormone is produced, the body sends a message back to the brain and pituitary centers to slow down. This is what happens when the system is functioning properly. However, this is not always the case. Some people experience a dysfunction in this system that can occur on multiple levels, including the hypothalamus (TRH production), pituitary gland (TSH production), or the thyroid gland (T4 and T3 production). Too much thyroid hormone production is called *hyperthyroidism* and is associated with weight loss and other symptoms of excessive metabolism, including racing heart, nervousness, and diarrhea. The most common condition is decreased thyroid hormone production or *hypothyroidism*, which is associated with weight gain. Other common symptoms that occur with hypothyroidism include: fatigue, feeling cold, low body temperature, dry skin, thinning hair, brittle nails, depression, poor memory and concentration, headaches, constipation, as well as others. Your healthcare provider can obtain a thyroid panel to make sure you have no abnormalities. There are also cases when the TSH and T4 levels appear normal, thus indicating a normal thyroid function. However, a person is still experiencing symptoms of hypothyroidism, including weight gain. This condition is known as Low T3 Syndrome. Therefore, even if TSH is normal, but you're still having symptoms of low thyroid, it may be worthwhile to check the Free T3 levels.

Cushing's syndrome: Also called hypercortisolism, this is a condition of too much corticosteroid production. This is usually the result of pituitary gland (site of normal production of ACTH) activity or other sites with tumors producing ACTH. Symptoms usually include obesity, excessive body hair, menstrual irregularities, muscle weakness or pains, skin conditions (including acne), bruising, swelling of the extremities, congestive heart failure, and frequent urination. Diagnosis is usually made at a physician's office following a work-up.

Prolactinoma: This is another pituitary tumor that causes excessive prolactin release. In women, it is associated with menstrual irregularities, infertility, and excessive galactorrhea (breast milk production). In men, it is associated with impotence and decreased libido, as well as other pituitary hormone problems due to the space occupying nature of this condition. Blood tests can detect increased prolactin levels and an MRI of the brain can detect the tumor's size. Treatment consists of medications in addition to a surgical resection.

Polycystic Ovarian Syndrome (PCOS) is a very common obesity-related condition in women and is associated with infertility, menstrual irregularities, increased body hair, as well as endometrial and breast cancer, diabetes, heart disease, and insulin resistance syndrome. Most common hormonal abnormalities include LH elevation (leutenizing hormone) in addition to increased estrogen (female sex hormones) and androgens (male sex hormones). This is usually confirmed by an ultrasound of the ovaries that shows multiple cysts and increased ovarian size.

Insulin Resistance Syndrome: This is present in up to a quarter of the population. It is an endocrine (metabolic) condition with genetic and environmental contributions. It is due to insulin's failure to move blood glucose (sugar) into cells, resulting in high insulin levels in response to food (especially carbohydrates) and leading into adult onset diabetes. Its presence is strongly associated with obesity and being overweight. This condition is largely due to extra weight, and, in turn, causes further obesity and weight gain that is difficult to treat. Having insulin resistance syndrome causes heart disease, hypertension, diabetes, stroke, high cholesterol, sleep apnea and multiple other conditions that have a common link with diabetes. There is a genetic component, or predisposition (like loading the gun), and environmental (lifestyle) factors (like pulling the trigger). Diagnosis is made by monitoring sugar levels and HgA1c (long term measure of sugar levels), or insulin levels. The definition of insulin resistance includes three or more of the following: (1) abdominal circumference of more than 40 inches in men or 35 in women; (2) triglycerides of more than 150 mg/dl; (3) HDL (good cholesterol) less than 40 in men and 50 in women; (4) blood pressure of greater than 130/85; and (5) fasting glucose of greater than 100. Treatment includes a proper diet (lower carbohydrate) and medications, including Metformin (serves to sensitize the body to the effect of insulin).

Diabetes (type 2, or adult onset): This is similar to insulin resistance in their biochemical causes, but it presents more obvious sugar level abnormalities. Diabetes and obesity have long had a relationship, and each contributes to the other. Obesity is a major risk factor for diabetes mellitus (DM) and most of the adult onset diabetics are overweight or obese. Presence of diabetes is a major risk factor in developing heart disease, among other problems, and includes the following complications: atherosclerosis (clogging of the blood vessels with cholesterol, thus decreasing blood circulation), heart disease, stroke, retinopathy (vision problems), nephropathy (kidney disease), and neuropathy (including pain and loss of sensation of feet and legs). The treatment for diabetes is initially diet and lifestyle changes. Weight loss is the single most effective way to reverse and prevent this condition. If this is not done, medications are usually prescribed. Some may help with weight loss while helping to control the sugar level, and others may contribute further to weight gain (see next chapter on common medications and their effect on weight).

Other common conditions, such as headaches, high blood pressure, and psychiatric disorders, require treatment with medications that tend to cause weight gain. If you are having difficultly losing weight while staying with a proper diet and exercise program, you may need to discuss your medication regimen with your doctor.

Personal Worksheets for Medications and Medical Problems

Do you have any medical problems such as diabetes, high blood pressure, thyroid, or any others that may affect your weight?

Do you take any regular medications?

If the answer is yes to either or both, make sure to make an appointment with your healthcare provider to discuss these issues; and see if there are any changes that can be made to help you with weight loss or to avoid weight gain.

If you are a diabetic taking medications, have high blood pressure (especially if taking a diuretic – water pill) or have other significant medical problems or medications, you may want to check with your doctor about modifying and/or monitoring the dose of medications along with the progression of the condition.

Often, with significant weight loss, the need for medications lessens, and maintaining the same doses will cause low blood sugar or low blood pressure, and thus the symptoms of such (example: dizziness, palpitations, etc…).

CHAPTER 9

Weight Loss Medications

Medications are also available specifically for the purpose of weight loss. The ones physicians prescribe generally fall into several categories: *appetite suppressors, fat absorption blockers*, and others that work by different mechanisms. Before proceeding with this option, be sure your healthcare provider is comfortable and familiar with the use of weight loss medications and that you understand the risks, benefits and directions for use of a particular medication.

Of note, children over 12 years old can qualify for fat absorption blockers, and children over the age of 16 can qualify for appetite suppressants if they fit the criteria. However, always keep in mind both your and your healthcare provider's level of comfort with the medications prior to initiating any course of treatment.

Appetite suppressors include Phentermine and FDA approved Meridia. In general, keep in mind that while they are generally safe for most people, certain conditions preclude their use. Some conditions with which they cannot be used are extremely high blood pressure that is not controlled well, significant heart disease, significant seizure activity, or if certain other medications are being used at the same time. Also, while taking this type of medication, it is important to regularly follow-up with your healthcare provider to monitor any intense symptoms or elevation in the blood pressure. The more common side effects frequently encountered are a slight elevation of heart rate, difficulty sleeping or feeling a little shaky. In the absence of other problems, these are relatively minor and tend to resolve on their own or can be treated with other medications.

Some people will respond very well to these medications, allowing them to reduce their caloric intake while keeping their appetite under control. Other people may not experience any significant effects. If you have tried such a medication without any progress for one to two months, it is likely not going to work for you. Another appetite suppressant may work instead, as the different medications work by affecting different pathways in the central nervous system and the brain.

In my practice, I often see people who are interested in "a pill" that will solve their weight problems. After a careful screening process that covers their medical history, diet, activity level, and lifestyle factors, I always advise them that while the pills may be helpful, especially during the diet, they are not by any means a "magic bullet." Even for those who do well with them, no weight loss will occur unless one changes the diet and activity levels. Also, if one is to rely on diet pills as "a magic bullet," as soon as they stop taking them, the weight comes right back. Furthermore, staying on the pills for the rest of one's life is unlikely, so the lifestyle changes are still essential to maintaining the progress over the long term.

Fat absorption blockers, such as Orlistat, work by preventing the absorption of fat in the gastrointestinal system. The idea is that fats have the highest caloric density of all the macronutrients at 9 calories per gram, while carbohydrates and proteins are only 4 calories per gram. These medications work best in combination with a low fat diet, and may serve as a way to discourage consumption of high fat content food. When a person taking Orlistat does have a fatty meal, the unabsorbed fats will pass into the stool, and thus the unpleasant side effects of abdominal discomfort, cramping and foul-smelling, loose stools.

The FDA approved, over-the-counter version can be found in *ALLI*, a fat absorption blocker that is half the dose of physician prescribed *Orlistat*. The package usually comes with general lifestyle and dietary advice, which is a great aspect of it. However, these medications are hardly what you would think of as a "magic bullet" either. Weight loss is usually moderate, losing only a few pounds more than with a diet alone. The side effects, as we discussed, make tolerating this medication difficult — unless one enjoys having those kinds of symptoms. Most of my clients have had a hard time staying with these medications even though the potential for moderate benefit does exist.

Other over-the-counter weight loss medications are quite plentiful and widely advertised. Most claim to be effective for weight loss. Walking through the aisles of pharmacies and grocery stores, I see no shortage of them; and every once in a while, one or two new brands appear. The same applies with infomercials on TV and other mediums. The one thing to realize is that, for the most part, they have not been tested, approved or regulated by the FDA; and they may or may not be safe and/or even effective. I have come to understand that just because something is labeled as "natural," "doctor recommended," or the like does not make it safe or effective. On the contrary, most of the prescription medications used today derived from "natural" sources and underwent a complicated and cumbersome FDA testing and approval process. Without being judgmental or making undue generalizations about all over-the-counter products, I suggest dieters to be very cautious with their use. In particular, be wary of the ones that sound like a "magic bullet" and minimize the importance of a healthy lifestyle. **If the claim sounds too good to be true, it probably is. If in doubt, check with your healthcare provider before purchasing or using any over-the-counter weight loss product**. You may be surprised to find some of them in medical references.

Personal Worksheet for Weight Loss Medications

What are your expectations and experiences with weight loss medications so far? (If you are considering using medications to help you with weight loss, make sure you have realistic expectations.)

Are you taking any over-the-counter weight loss medications currently? If so, please make sure to check with your healthcare provider or a local pharmacy about the safety and any possible known interactions with other medications.

If you are considering a prescription weight loss medication, check with your healthcare provider about his or her comfort and recommendations.

CHAPTER 10

Weight Loss Surgery

This chapter will review the basic principles behind weight loss surgery although it does not claim, in any way, to be a complete and comprehensive source of information. Your healthcare provider and the internet both provide a useful source of information about these procedures.

Bariatric surgery (from the Greek words "baros" meaning "weight," and "iatrikos" meaning "medicine") is the collective term for a group of surgical procedures that may be used to promote weight loss in certain cases. Surgical procedures are recommended ONLY for those with severe obesity who have not responded to diet, exercise, or medication. For those with less severe obesity, the risks of the surgical procedure may outweigh any potential benefits. Candidates should be sure they understand the implications of bariatric surgery and are willing to commit to the lifestyle changes necessary for reaching and maintaining a healthy weight following the procedure.

The National Institutes of Health recommends that surgery be considered for people at the following weight levels:

- Patients with a body mass index > 40

(see Appendix C to calculate your BMI)

- Patients with a body mass index between 35 and 40 who also have serious medical problems (diabetes, high blood pressure, disabling joint conditions such as arthritis, or obstructive sleep apnea) that would improve with weight loss

Preparing for Surgery

Most patients in the United States who undergo a weight loss surgery must meet with several healthcare providers before surgery is scheduled. This often includes a nutritionist and mental health specialist. The nutritionist ensures that the patient understands and can follow the strict dietary guidelines necessary after surgery. Some patients will be required to lose a small amount of weight before surgery. The mental health specialist helps the patient to identify factors involved in stress, coping and lifestyle. Some patients need to work with these providers for several weeks or months before proceeding with surgery.

Other healthcare providers may also be involved in the pre-surgical evaluation, including a cardiologist, internal medicine specialist, or sleep medicine specialist. A cardiologist helps to ensure that the patient's heart is healthy enough for surgery. An internal medicine provider may be needed to assess the patient's overall health. A sleep medicine specialist can determine if the patient has a common obesity-related condition called sleep apnea. Sleep apnea can cause difficulty breathing while sleeping and may pose a risk around the time of surgery.

Types of Surgeries

Weight-loss surgery can be divided into the following categories: restrictive, mal-absorptive, and mixed or combination. A comparison of these procedures is available in Table 2 on page 100. All of these procedures are performed under general anesthesia (the patient is given medication to induce sleep).

Restrictive: Restrictive procedures reduce the size of the stomach, limiting the amount of food that can be consumed at once. There are several types of restrictive surgeries.

Mal-absorptive: In the normal digestive process, food is swallowed and then enters the stomach. It is then pushed into the small intestine and is mixed with digestive juices and bile. Throughout the long loops of the small intestine, the intestinal walls absorb nutrients (vitamins, carbohydrates, proteins, and fats) from the food. The remaining contents are then passed into the large intestine, where water is absorbed, and then out of the body in the form of feces.

The goal of mal-absorptive surgical procedures is to have food bypass the small intestine, thereby reducing the absorption of calories and inducing weight loss. Biliopancreatic diversion, with or without duodenal switch (taking the upper part of the small intestine and reconnecting it to the lower portion instead), is the primary mal-absorptive procedure performed today.

Mixed: Mixed or combination procedures have both a restrictive and mal-absorptive component, meaning that they limit food intake while also decreasing absorption of nutrients within the body. A gastric bypass is the most common mixed surgical procedure used to treat weight loss in the United States.

Although bariatric surgery can produce dramatic results, it is crucial that the patient make a commitment to maintaining a healthy lifestyle, including follow-up contact with a healthcare provider to monitor progress. It can be difficult to make lifestyle adjustments after weight-loss surgery, and patients should be aware that they will have to work to develop and stick to new habits.

Table 2 (Source: AATCO)

Category	Restrictive and Malabsorptive (stomach and intestines)		Restrictive (stomach only)	
Operation	Roux-en-Y Gastric Bypass Surgery	Vertical Gastrectomy with Duodenal Switch	Vertical Sleeve Gastrectomy	Lap-Band Procedure
Procedure	Small 1 ounce pouch connected to the small intestine.	Long vertical pouch measuring about 4-5 oz. The duodenum is connected to the last 6 feet of small intestine.	Long narrow vertical pouch measuring 2-3 oz. Identical to the duodenal switch pouch but smaller.	An adjustable silicone band is placed around the top part of the stomach creating a small 1-2 ounce pouch.
Function	Significantly restricts the volume of food that can be consumed.	Moderately restricts the volume of food that can be consumed.	Significantly restricts the volume of food that can be consumed.	Moderately restricts the volume and type of foods able to be eaten. Creates sensation of fullness
Weight Loss	70% loss of excess weight. More failures (loss of <50% excess weight) than the DS.	80% excess weight loss. More patients lose too much weight or develop nutritional problems than the RNY.	60-70% excess weight loss.	60% excess weight loss. Requires the most dietary and exercise effort of all procedures.
Recovery Time	2-3 weeks	2-3 weeks	1-2 weeks	1 week
Common Use	Patients with a BMI of 35-55 kg/m2 and those with a "sweet-tooth."	Patients with a BMI of > 50 kg/m2. Those with BMI of <45 kg/m2 may lose too much weight.	High risk or very heavy (BMI > 60 kg/m2) patients as a "first-stage" procedure.	Patients who enjoy exercising and are more disciplined in following dietary restrictions.
Possible Side Effects	Dumping syndrome Ulcers Bowel obstruction Anemia Vitamin/Mineral deficiencies Leak	Nausea and vomiting Heartburn Severe diarrhea Kidney stones Ulcers Bowel obstruction Nutritional/Vitamin deficiencies Loss of too much weight requiring reoperation Leak	Nausea and vomiting Heartburn Inadequate weight loss Weight regain Additional procedure may be needed to obtain adequate weight loss Leak	Slow weight loss Slippage Erosion Infection Port problems Device malfunction

Personal Worksheet for Weight Loss Surgery

What are your feelings about weight loss surgery, and do you consider this an option for you? If yes, answer the following questions below:

Do I qualify for weight loss surgery? Using the BMI calculation (if not sure, ask your healthcare provider), determine if are you at body mass index of 40, or 35 with medical problems such as diabetes, high blood pressure. If in doubt, check with your local hospital or ASBS.org for local resources on bariatric surgery and further information.

If you do want to explore the weight loss surgery as an option, are you ready to commit to lifestyle changes that are required to make the surgery work for you? If so, what changes are you willing to make now?

CHAPTER 11

Maintaining Your Progress

Maintaining your progress is the most important part of the process once you've lost the weight or are close to achieving your desired weight. Most people will have no problems losing some amount of weight only to fall into a "Yo-Yo" pattern of weight loss and regain. The regain is usually even more than the original starting weight for most people as they slip into their old habits. One reason is that if weight loss is not done in a balanced fashion without any increase in the physical activity, the lean body mass (muscle) is also lost together with the fat mass. Even under the ideal conditions, at least 25 percent of the weight lost will be the lean body (muscle) loss. Under less than ideal conditions, especially with fad or starvation diets, the lean body weight loss will be greater. This has the effect of lowering the metabolic rate (the rate at which the body burns calories). Thus, if a person goes back to their prior caloric intake, now the calories incoming are even greater in proportion to the calories being expended. This creates a significant positive caloric imbalance (more incoming than outgoing), resulting in weight gain. Therefore, during the weight maintenance phase, all your prior hard work at changing lifestyle habits, increasing activity and exercise levels, and monitoring your caloric intake become essential.

Recommendations for Adults

Typical caloric weight maintenance requirements for men are 2,300 to 2,900 calories/day and for women 1,900 to 2,200 calories/day. A rough formula for calculating the calories to maintain the weight is the following:

Male: 12 x weight in lbs x activity factor

Female: 11 x weight in lbs x activity factor

Activity factor is as follows:

- Sedentary: 1.2
- Three aerobic events per week: 1.3
- Five aerobic events per week: 1.5
- Seven aerobic events per week: 1.6
- Endurance athletic training: 1.7

Although there are ways to calculate energy expenditure using technology, the simplest way is to observe what happens to you with your current lifestyle and eating habits. If you are gaining weight, then this needs to be addressed. If you are feeling good and either losing or maintaining your weight at your desired level, then you are doing something right.

Be aware that during the maintenance phase of weight control, the weight will vary, especially for women. This has to do with salt and water retention, hormonal changes, and the different phases of the menstrual cycle. It is not unusual to see variations of up to three to four pounds, even during the course of a single day. This does not mean that you have gained weight. However, a weight regain of more than three to four pounds that is persisting, generally should not be attributed to water retention or any other transient effect. Instead, use it as an alarm that something about your diet, lifestyle and the caloric balance has changed, and weight is being regained. After regaining just a few pounds is a good time to get a handle on this once more by paying attention to your diet, activity and lifestyle factors. This is also a good time to visit your healthcare provider if you suspect that there may be something else happening, such as a medical condition, a change in medication or another issue.

It has been said that the only thing that is constant in our lives is change. By being aware, proactive and going back to the tools utilized during the active weight loss process, the transient weight gain will not become permanent and will remain within your control. I cannot emphasize enough that this is the most important thing to understand and keep in mind: losing weight is *only* a part of the picture. **Weight control is the ultimate goal**, and it does require adjustment of all of the above mentioned factors, including lifestyle, diet and exercise.

For people who have ever struggled with their weight, the following information will be particularly interesting. In the United States, an official study keeps track of those individuals who have lost a significant amount of weight and have been able to keep it off successfully. The common characteristics of these individuals are summarized in the *National Weight Control Registry* and include:

- Eating a daily breakfast
- Self-monitoring, including a food and exercise diary and daily weight monitoring
- Exercise to burn at least 400 calories per day for an average of 3-5 days per week
- Realistic goal-setting
- Good stress tolerance and coping mechanisms
- A strong social support system, including friends and family

As far as the composition of nutrition for weight maintenance, it should be balanced in both micronutrients and macronutrients. In the vast literature available on maintenance diets, there is no one definitive standard to advocate. In general, keeping the diet balanced, healthy, high in fiber and rich in vitamins and minerals will do the job. As previously stated, try to keep an approximate ratio of: proteins at or above 30 percent (lean preferred); fats 5 to 30 percent (limiting saturated, trans-fats and cholesterol); and carbohydrates not exceeding 50 percent (limiting simple sugars and increasing the amount of complex starches, including high fiber, whole wheat/grain enriched products). A complete multi-vitamin supplement (A-Z) is usually sufficient given a balanced diet together with fish oil or Omega 3 and 6 supplements. (Taking mega doses is usually not recommended and is potentially harmful.) Please see the Appendix I for the guidelines for 1,600 to 3,200 calorie balanced maintenance diets. Most importantly, each person has a distinct interaction of genetic, environmental and social factors. Thus, no one particular diet or exercise pattern will work for everyone in the same way. You should use these guidelines as general starting points and adjust the diet and activity pattern to fit your particular situation and needs.

Recommendations for Children and Adolescents

When it comes to children and adolescents, the principles mentioned above still apply. However, special considerations, which are listed below, exist. The important definitions regarding childhood weight categories based on pediatric charts are:

> **At Risk of Overweight**: Body mass index for age (BMI-for-age) between 85 and 95 percent for ages 2 to 20 years old.
>
> **Overweight**: BMI-for-age at or above 95 percent for ages 2 to 20 years old.

Up to 2 years old: healthcare providers and parents can still use weight-for-age charts, and keep a close eye on the progress over time.

For children over 2 years old, the BMI-for-age or weight-for-stature charts should be utilized. (Please see the appendix section for the charts mentioned here, and feel free to consult with your healthcare provider for further questions.)

For children especially, maintenance of weight plays an important part, not only after reaching the desired weight, but also as an active weight loss process itself in a growing child. Children and adolescents have something in their favor that adults lack. That something is physical growth and development. Every inch of growth is equivalent to five pounds of weight loss if the weight is maintained during the growth stages. Thus, a child who grew by two inches but maintained the same weight would have lost about ten pounds.

The general recommendations for weight maintenance as a weight loss tool for children and adolescents are:

0-2 years: Monitor the growth curves.

2-7 years at-risk-for-overweight or overweight without medical complications: Weight maintenance or, in other words, maintaining the current weight while the child is growing.

7 years old or older at-risk-for-overweight without medical complications: Weight maintenance as mentioned above.

Family therapy with parents is just as important in the weight loss process, especially with the focus on the person responsible for the child's food. Another factor well worth mentioning is family communication and relationships. When the child is less than 6 years of age, parental influence and factors matter most. Over 6 years of age, a child's, especially an adolescent's, individual choices and actions start to come into play and become more significant.

Physical activity is important and at least one hour per day is recommended. For those who are sedentary, any increase is highly recommended. At the same time, a reduction in television, video games, computer-based activities, as well as other sedentary activities, should be limited to less than one to two hours per day.

Taking into account age, sex and activity level, the following table describes in more detail the usual caloric requirements to maintain the weight:

Average Maintenance Needs for Children:

Age	Female Sedentary	30-60 min/d	>60 min/d	Male Sedentary	30-60 min/d	>60 min/d
2	1000	1000	1000	1000	1000	1000
3	1000	1200	1400	1000	1400	1400
4	1200	1400	1400	1200	1400	1600
5	1200	1400	1600	1200	1400	1600
6	1200	1400	1600	1400	1600	1800
7	1200	1600	1800	1400	1600	1800
8	1400	1600	1800	1400	1600	2000
9	1400	1600	1800	1600	1800	2000
10	1400	1800	2000	1600	1800	2200
11	1600	1800	2000	1800	2000	2200
12	1600	2000	2200	1800	2200	2400
13	1600	2000	2200	2000	2200	2600
14	1800	2000	2400	2000	2400	2800
15	1800	2000	2400	2200	2600	3000
16	1800	2000	2400	2400	2800	3200
17	1800	2000	2400	2400	2800	3200
18	1800	2000	2400	2400	2800	3200

Note: Females 14 and up are about adult level; males 16 and up are about adult level. (Source: http://www.mypyramid.gov)

Based on the recommended caloric level, see the appendices for dietary guidelines for balanced pediatric and adolescent maintenance programs.

Personal Worksheet for Weight Loss Maintenance

What are your feelings or experiences thus far about a lifelong process of weight control?

What weight loss and/or maintenance have you achieved in the past that you can learn from, and how can you turn that into a lesson and long-term motivation?

What strengths or techniques do you have now that you can utilize and put into practice when needed?

How can you use your higher power to keep on track in difficult situations or during "lapse" periods?

CHAPTER 12

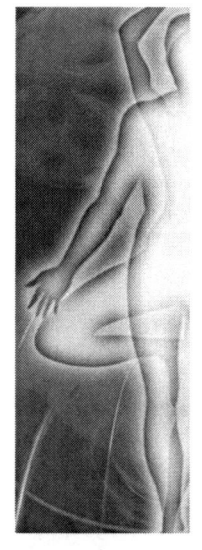

Power Principle Summary

Medical science in the field of nutrition and weight loss invariably progresses and changes over time. Popular diets will come and go and, likely, be recycled under new names and marketing strategies, touting "new and improved," "quick and easy," "natural," and so forth.

As medical science advances, new diet, nutrition and weight loss information will appear, and some things that we take for granted will become obsolete. The greatest progress to be made is likely in the field of genetics. Each and every individual is different, and when scientists are able to tap into a particular individual's genetic predisposition to customize a wellness and weight loss program, the results will be phenomenal. Also, with more developments on the molecular level and cellular function, products that affect metabolism and basic human functioning are likely to emerge as well.

Like a gun that can be used to protect or to cause harm, we too have the power to determine which direction our life, health and weight will take. The majority of the book has focused on the body aspect, including nutrition, exercise, activity, lifestyle, and the current state of the medical science as it relates to weight. This body aspect directly determines what we see in a mirror and the numbers we see on a scale. However, this aspect is constantly undergoing major changes and will likely continue to do so. Therefore, it is important to keep up with new developments as they surface, including accurate information (both dietary and medical), as well as new tools, such as medications, supplements, equipment, and diet plans. These are all great tools, but they are only useful in the hands of the one who chooses to use them.

The other aspects of weight control that are more enduring and powerful are the mind and spirit. The mind aspect includes knowledge, attitudes, and goals. It directs and drives the body aspects mentioned above. It is not immune to sickness, weakness and misdirection. Meanwhile, it has the capacity to lead to success even in the most difficult circumstances, and it has the capacity of rendering failure even when we are physically able of achieving success. The Power Principle addresses the latter, most important aspect, but it also goes further than that in addressing the spirit.

The spirit aspect of the Power Principle is its final and most significant component. Once the Spirit-Mind-Body axis is properly aligned, the spirit will guide the mind in the right direction, and the mind will in turn lead to body (physical) changes. Furthermore, the spirit will serve as the lighthouse for the mind even in the stormiest of weather, and it will help to put it back on the right course no matter what takes place or where you are in life.

A principle in Buddhism speaks of enlightenment, a state where one reaches a higher spiritual ground and understanding. One way in which this can be represented is the following: a person's journey starts on one bank of the river (the starting, un-enlightened point) with the goal of reaching the other bank of the river, where the state of enlightenment can be achieved. In the process, the raft that one takes to cross the river can be thought of as the principles and practices of Buddhism. It is said that once one reaches the other side of the river and looks back over the river and onto the bank of the river from where the journey started, the enlightened realizes a simple, but powerful truth. The capacity of being and feeling enlightened has always been there within, no matter what bank of the river one is on, and it is simply a matter of acknowledging that state and allowing oneself to be in it. In essence, the experience of enlightenment can then be recreated and obtained at a moment's notice as one desires and allows it.

The Power Principle, the power to know yourself, to change yourself and to move yourself in the direction of improvement, whether it relates to weight or anything else of importance, once realized and obtained, is always there with you. As our busy lives get busier and unforeseen events take place, losing track of our inner self becomes easy. However, remember your true priorities, and the fact that you have the power to act on them. Reach within and bring back that power. It is yours always.

APPENDICES

Appendices

A. Terms Related to Energy (Calorie) Expenditure

Calorie (same as Kilocalorie): The amount of heat/energy necessary to raise 1 kilogram of water by 1 degree Celsius.

Resting Metabolic Rate (RMR): Energy expended by the body during the resting state for the purpose of maintaining basic body functions. It correlates with gender (women are lower), lean body mass, slight decline with age, and body temperature (more with more warmth). This constitutes the largest component of energy needs (about 60 to 70 percent on average in a moderately active individual).

Resting Energy Expenditure (REE): A term for energy at rest or in ambient conditions (not necessarily in bed). It is used by the World Health Organization and differs less than 10 percent from RMR. In clinical practice and daily life, it is used interchangeably with RMR.

Physical Activity: Involves being in motion or active throughout the day. Though considered as a normal human function, it significantly contributes to calorie burning. One measure of this is via the use of a pedometer.

Exercise: A formal, purposeful bodily activity to improve the fitness level and overall health. This is done in addition to the physical activity of daily living and is an essential aspect of weight control.

Voluntary Energy Expenditure: Can amount to up to 20 to 40 percent of energy expenditure in a fairly active individual. In general, this factor has declined significantly due to the sedentary lifestyles of both adults and children.

Other determinants of energy needs:
Age: Lean body mass tends to decline beyond early adulthood at two to three percent per decade.

Gender: Men tend to have more lean body mass than women, thus about 10 percent difference in REE.

Growth: Except for first year of life, it is typically a small component (see pediatric weight loss and maintenance chapters).

Body size: The larger the body size, the more energy per unit of time is expanded for any given activity, but more closely related to lean body mass than total body mass.

Climate: Caloric usage increases in extreme heat as well as in cold exposure (due to increased muscle activity or shivering).

Pregnancy: Increases need by about 300 Cal/day.

Lactation: Increases need by about 500 Cal/day

B. *Diet and Nutrition Basics*

MACRONUTRIENTS provide sources of calories to support the body's functions and voluntary activity. Unlike micronutrients, the body needs them in large quantities. They include proteins, carbohydrates, fats and water.

Proteins

Recommended Daily Allowance (RDA) amounts are about 1 gm/kg/day. For an average person, the amount should be able to maintain lean body mass, especially during a period of dieting or a reduced calorie intake. This equates to the following: men - 63 gm/day and women - 50 gm/day. When on either maintenance or regular diet, the recommended amount of calories from proteins should be equal to or more than 30 percent. Proteins furnish amino acids required to build and maintain body tissues. The energy source equivalent of proteins is 4 cal/gm.

Dietary sources: Meat, poultry, fish, milk, legumes (soybeans, peanuts, peas, beans, lentils). They may also be found in some cereals (but in smaller amounts).

Requirements are based on maintenance of nitrogen balance: the difference between nitrogen intake (via amino acids) and the amount excreted in urine, feces, sweat and other losses. During periods of growth, the balance must be in the positive (more intake than excretion) to allow for formation of new tissue.

Essential **amino acids** cannot be made by the body and must be consumed in the daily diet. They include the following: leucine, isoleucine, valine, tryptophan, phenylalanine, methionine, threonine, lysine, and histidine (in infants only; adults have the ability to synthesize it).

Deficiency is rare as an isolated condition. When it does occur, it is usually in conjunction with energy and other nutrient deficiencies from either insufficient food intake, an unbalanced diet or due to illness.

Excess: No current firm evidence exists that increased levels are harmful, other than consuming more than required for optimal functioning and with the body metabolizing the extra protein into fat. For some people who have kidney problems, it is advisable to check with their doctor before initiating a high protein diet.

Effect on dieting and weight management: High protein diets can be an important part of maintaining satiety, increasing thermo-genesis (calorie consumption), and protection of lean body mass (especially in periods of dieting and reduced overall caloric intake). When on maintenance (at or above 1,500 calorie level), it is usually sufficient to keep protein calories at or above 30 percent of overall caloric intake. During dieting or reduced caloric intake, the amount of protein calories needs to be greater.

Carbohydrates

Carbohydrates are the most abundant source of calories in the typical western culture. They are a source of much controversy with regard to their effect on the diet, and limiting the amount consumed is the principle behind many popular diets, as well as a source of many discussions among healthcare professionals.

RDA amounts: The classical recommendation with a 2,000 calorie diet is about 50 percent of overall calories or 250 gm/day. The energy content is 4 cal/gm.

Sources include dairy (milk, cheese, yogurt, etc...); grains (breads, rice); sweets; fruits; certain vegetables (i.e. potatoes, carrots, etc...)

Types of carbohydrates: They can be classified as simple (sugars), or complex (starches), which contain a significant source of dietary fiber, especially in fruits and vegetables (soluble fiber); insoluble fiber (cellulose and some hemi-cellulose), ex: bran layer of cereals.

Deficiency: Usually there are no significant problems with limiting or eliminating carbohydrates, assuming the rest of the diet is fairly balanced. There is no minimum defined amount or essential nutrients that can't be generated or replaced by the body. However, one must be aware of dietary fiber deficiency, which can lead to constipation and possible connection to colon cancer (with long term deficiency).

Excess is the most common problem facing the western societies, and now more than ever, developing societies as well. Being that carbohydrates are the most abundant and least expensive source of calories available, they are being consumed in far greater proportion than any other macronutrient and marketed, often inappropriately, by the food manufacturing companies as the recommended staple food.

Effect on dieting and weight management: There is and has long been a controversy regarding the role and effects of carbohydrates on weight control. There is a school of thought that it is the overall calorie balance that matters and not the composition of the diet. Thus, according to this theory, as long as one's intake of calories is less than what is being burned or utilized by the body, weight loss will occur regardless of what one is eating.

This theory has been challenged in a public fashion since mid-19th century, with emergence of low carbohydrate diets. This trend has continued with the popular low carbohydrate diets including Atkins, Ornish, South Beach; many commercial programs, and individually designed physician- and/or dietician-based programs. While the controversy still continues, within bariatric (weight loss) medicine research, a pattern is emerging that supports the theory that there is a role for monitoring diet content, and not only the amount of calories.

Glycemic Index: With regards to carbohydrates, the latest trend (and with mounting evidence behind it) is that the *glycemic index* of the carbohydrates does matter with regard to effect on weight control. There is even further evidence that most people who are overweight or obese are likely insulin-resistant, if not overtly diabetic. The role of insulin (which usually functions to utilize the sugar in the bloodstream for energy needs) has taken a central role. Those who are insulin resistant or diabetic, release a lot of insulin, which in turn has a difficult time utilizing the existing blood sugars. The more insulin in the bloodstream, and the higher sugar level, the more the hunger and fatigue one feels; and this often leads to more food and calorie intake. Last but not least, with insulin resistance, there is the effect of converting sugars into the storage form of fat instead of effective utilization as the energy source.

Foods that have *high glycemic index* (cause a stronger insulin release), especially simple carbohydrates or sugars, tend to magnify this effect with the cycle of worsening obesity and low energy levels. Foods that have *low glycemic index* (usually complicated, whole grain, and high fiber sources of carbohydrates) are better tolerated and do not induce as much of the insulin response. These generally tend to be healthier options for carbohydrates, and while on maintenance phase of weight control, should be 50 percent or greater of the overall carbohydrates consumed. When on a calorie-restrictive diet, the amount of carbohydrates should be adjusted appropriately, especially depending on the caloric level and the type of the diet. It is not unusual to completely eliminate carbohydrates altogether for a time period up to a number of weeks in order to jump-start the process, as is currently utilized in Atkins diet, Phase 1 of the South Beach diet, as well as other diets, including those custom-designed by health professionals. As the time goes on, it is generally recommended to incorporate carbohydrates back into the diet. The choice of carbohydrates to be introduced into the diet should take into account their nutritional value, glycemic index, fiber, vitamins and mineral composition as well as other factors.

Other controversies surrounding carbohydrates. **High-fructose corn syrup** has been and is widely being used by food processing companies to improve the taste of both solid foods and drinks. It is currently being investigated for its effect on the liver glucose metabolism, in particular, the glucose uptake pathways. One possibility is the resulting increased fatty and triglyceride synthesis, which may lead to worsening of or induction of insulin resistance and metabolic syndrome.

Lipids/Fats

The caloric amount of fats is the highest (densest) of all the macronutrients, at 9 cal/gm. The **role of fats** is to aid in the transport and absorption of the fat soluble vitamins, and slowing down the transition of food via the stomach. Other effects are to increase the palatability of food and to increase the feelings of satiety.

Dietary sources include the animal sources, especially beef and fish, and plant oils (nuts and vegetables).

RDA amounts, based on a 2,000 calorie diet, should range between 5 to 30 percent of calories. The upper limit with this recommendation is not to exceed 67 grams (given the very caloric density).

Sub-categories: As far as nutrition, it is necessary to consider fats for their saturation factor which is a measure of its effect on blood vessels and other health effects. In general, the more *unsaturated*, the healthier the fat, and the more likely it is to be liquid (ex: olive oil). The more *saturated* it is, the more artery clogging its capability, and generally tends to be solid (ex: butter). As far as national recommendations, it is advised to keep saturated fatty acids to less that 10 percent of daily calories.

Trans-fat is yet another category, which has come under increased attention and monitoring in recent years. Trans-fat is not a natural fat; rather, it is an invention by the food processing companies to increase the shelf life of products and to maintain fats in the solid form for a significant amount of time. They are readily found in sweets (cookies, cakes, etc ...) and a variety of other foods, including many fast foods. The evidence behind their obvious harmful effects on health, including heart disease, strokes, heart attacks and multiple others, is very clear. Other countries have banned their use altogether. It is still legal in the United States, but since 2006, legislation has passed, requiring food manufacturers to include this information on food labels. It is still up to the consumer to read those labels and to decide for themselves how to go about this issue. While the ideal situation is to completely eliminate foods that contain trans-fats, simply limiting their amounts in a diet will go a long way to a healthier lifestyle.

Essential Fatty Acids: There are 2 fatty acids that cannot be synthesized by humans which are essential for body function as well as carrying fat soluble vitamins. They are linolenic acid (Omega-6 fatty acid), and alpha-linolenic acid (Omega-3 fatty acid).

Deficiency: Linolenic acid deficiency causes poor growth and dermatitis (skin irritation/inflammation) among other problems. Alpha-linolenic acid is converted to hormone-like substances that reduce inflammation. Deficiency causes neurological changes (numbness, tingling, weakness, blurring of vision). While the deficiency is mostly related to the essential fatty acids, there are also possible deficiencies from lack of the fat-soluble vitamins (see Micronutrients section below).

Excess: Typical American diets have an excessive amount of fats, especially trans-fats and saturated fats, often in excess of 30 percent. Other than that, its effects are related to the high caloric density of fats (9 cal/gm), which contributes significantly to excess calories and, thus, excess fat storage in the body.

Effect on weight management: Prior to the current popularity of the low carbohydrate diets, it was the low fat diet that was encouraged for the benefit of weight loss. It is also the target of a prescription medication Orlistat (which eliminates up to 30 percent of fats from the digestive tract, and has been released in a nonprescription form as ALLI over the counter). The principle behind a low fat diet has to do with the high caloric density of fats (9 cal/gm). This principle still has a significant value when one is on a limited overall calorie diet. Problems with focusing only on the low-fat component is that it does not take into account the carbohydrate factor and the glycemic index (see above). Also, severely fat-reduced diets will often lack the palatability, and it is a known fact that unless one enjoys the food (at least to some degree), the diet is not likely to be maintained in the long term. The best way to approach fats when considering a diet is to make sure to incorporate the basic minimum amount to prevent a deficiency, try to maintain the quality of fats, (mostly unsaturated, less than 10 percent saturated, and to try to eliminate trans-fats as much as possible), and ensure that the fat-soluble vitamins are taken appropriately (see below). One guideline to stay with as far as a minimum amount in the diet is at or about 10 gm, which is easily present if one incorporates vegetables, and meat/poultry/fish (preferably lean, or low fat). It is important to understand that it is possible to have a calorie-reduced diet that has sufficient protein, low carbohydrates, low fat, and still be complete, balanced, and palatable.

Cholesterol is another substance that does not contribute much in terms of calories, yet is an essential component of cellular membranes, as well as a component of steroid hormones (including sex hormones), and bile acids. For a healthy individual, without significant cardiac risk factors or a history of elevated cholesterol, the recommended amount is less than 300 mg/day. If one does have significant health issues or any other concerns, it is recommended to reduce the amount to less than 200 mg/day, since high cholesterol is a risk factor for heart and vascular disease.

Alcohol: This is yet another source of calories and contributes significantly to the caloric intake. First, each gram of alcohol has 7 cal/gram, a number almost as significant as fats. However, unlike other macronutrients, it has no vitamins or minerals (see below), thus, it is often called "empty calories." It is not unusual for an alcoholic drink to contain up to several hundred calories. For example, a 5 oz glass of wine is 100 calories, a can of beer (12 oz) is 160 calories, and a mixed drink, such as a Margarita can be up to 270 calories. This number becomes significant when having more than one drink or having them often. The other way that alcohol contributes to caloric intake is by its un-inhibiting effect on the mind, causing one to eat more than one would, normally.

MICRONUTRIENTS include vitamins (fat-soluble and water-soluble), minerals, and trace elements. They are present in the body in small amounts but are essential for cellular and organ function, as well as the metabolism within the body.

Vitamins

Fat-soluble vitamins include vitamins A, D, E, and K, and these tend to accumulate in the body. Therefore, it is important not only to get an adequate amount, but to be aware of having too much, as they could be toxic.

Vitamin A plays a role in vision, skin, digestive and urinary body systems.

Vitamin D plays a role in bone and kidney function, among other systems. *Deficiency* results in bone problems such as osteoporosis and kidney problems. It is usually given with calcium supplementation and comes in prescription as well as over-the-counter varieties.

Vitamin E (alpha-tocopherol) is a significant factor in oxidation-reduction reactions and free radical binding. For that reason, it is thought of as having an anti-aging effect (though that has not been firmly established yet in medical sciences).

Vitamin K affects the body's ability to control bleeding. While taking this vitamin, you should be beware of its effect on coumadin (a blood thinning medication given to some patients with certain heart or stroke related conditions).

Water-soluble vitamins are usually excreted in the urine if too much is consumed. Thus, the term "expensive urine" is sometimes used when people take mega doses of these vitamins.

B1 (Thiamine) is involved in carbohydrate metabolism. *Deficiency* results in heart, brain and nervous system effects.

B2 (Riboflavin) is involved in energy production. *Deficiency* results in light sensitivity, salivation, sore lips and tongue.

B3 (Niacin) is involved in reduction-oxidation reactions in the body, as well as cholesterol treatment. *Deficiency* leads to a condition called Pellagra which is associated with the 4 D's (dermatitis, dementia, diarrhea, death) in addition to tremors, sore tongue. While there is no significant risk with taking Niacin, some people do experience side effect such as flushing (especially when used to treat cholesterol).

B6 (Pyridoxine) is involved in carbohydrate, fat and protein metabolism.

B12 (Cyanocobalamin) is usually given as a supplement to those with low levels manifested as a having anemia (pernicious type) or low blood levels of red blood cells. It is involved in blood cell formation, red blood cell maturation, and nucleic acid synthesis; it is absorbed in the distal ileum (distal part of the small bowel). *Deficiency* can lead to anemia (low blood count-see above), as well as having an effect on the nervous system.

Folic Acid is involved in blood cell maturation and infant development in pregnancy. Additionally, it is important for individual cell function, especially those that have a faster rate of turnover. *Deficiency* is associated with problems with rapidly dividing cells (blood cells, skin, digestive tract and others).

Biotin is involved in glucose and fatty acid (fats) metabolism. *Deficiency* results in skin and hair problems, and may also cause nausea.

B5 (Pantothenic Acid) is involved in certain metabolic reactions that the body requires, but there is no known deficiency for this particular vitamin.

Vitamin C (ascorbic acid) is involved in oxidation-reduction (free radical) reactions, carbohydrate, and protein metabolism, as well as immune system functioning. It is also, popularly regarded as having an anti-aging effect largely due to its effect on free radicals. *Deficiency* causes scurvy (i.e. bleeding gums historically seen with sailors on long voyages with limited dietary options). *Deficiency* may also result from mega-dose withdrawal (mega doses can be found with some vitamin formulations, in levels exceeding 1000 percent of the recommended amounts). This is yet another reason to be careful with vitamin supplements that contain mega doses of certain vitamins, even if they are water-soluble.

Vitamin like factors: Their role and requirements are unclear as far as their effect on the body and include *choline* and *carnitine*.

Minerals

Electrolytes (or minerals) to consider in diets include potassium, magnesium, phosphorus, and calcium. They contribute to various functions in the body, and a significant *deficiency or excess* may become life-threatening. If there is any question at all about the levels of electrolytes, it is very important to see a healthcare provider and have appropriate testing done.

Trace elements in diets are also of uncertain relationship with weight loss and include:

> **Chromium** regulates metabolism, is a co-factor for insulin, and has been marketed for weight loss; but there is no proven effect based on medical literature currently.
>
> **Vanadium** has a potential role in insulin resistance, but there also no proven effect based on medical literature at the current time.

Water

Water is the other essential component of the body, and having adequate hydration status is essential to good health. In general, it is recommended to drink 6 to 8 glasses per day or about 64 ounces. That number, however, is also dependant on personal medical history and individual circumstances. In general, it is a good idea to consult a healthcare provider, especially if you have heart, kidney or any other significant medical problems or simply are not sure.

C. Body Mass Index

The following table is from **www.cdc.gov** and can be used for adults to predict, in general terms, where your weight falls as far as being of normal weight for height, overweight, obese, or extremely obese. It does not, however, take into account the fact that muscle weighs more than fat. For this reason, athletes with larger amounts of muscle mass or those with a heavier bony structure may fall into the category of overweight, whereas they really are within normal limits or better than average as far as their body fat percentage. If, however, the weight for height falls into the category of obese or extremely obese, it is fairly accurate to say that the body fat percentage is greater than normal.

To calculate the Body Mass Index (BMI):

Start with your height;
Go horizontally across the table to find your current weight;
Follow the column where your weight is up to the top of the table to find the corresponding BMI.

For example: a person who's height is 5 foot 5 inches tall and weighs 160 pounds has a BMI between 26 and 27, a value that is in the overweight category.

Body Mass Index Table

BMI	19	20	21	22	23	24	25	26	27	28	29	30	31	32	33	34	35	36	37	38	39	40	41	42	43	44	45	46	47	48	49	50	51	52	53	54
	Normal						Overweight					Obese										Extreme Obesity														
Height (inches)												Body Weight (pounds)																								
58	91	96	100	105	110	115	119	124	129	134	138	143	148	153	158	162	167	172	177	181	186	191	196	201	205	210	215	220	224	229	234	239	244	248	253	258
59	94	99	104	109	114	119	124	128	133	138	143	148	153	158	163	168	173	178	183	188	193	198	203	208	212	217	222	227	232	237	242	247	252	257	262	267
60	97	102	107	112	118	123	128	133	138	143	148	153	158	163	168	174	179	184	189	194	199	204	209	215	220	225	230	235	240	245	250	255	261	266	271	276
61	100	106	111	116	122	127	132	137	143	148	153	158	164	169	174	180	185	190	195	201	206	211	217	222	227	232	238	243	248	254	259	264	269	275	280	285
62	104	109	115	120	126	131	136	142	147	153	158	164	169	175	180	186	191	196	202	207	213	218	224	229	235	240	246	251	256	262	267	273	278	284	289	295
63	107	113	118	124	130	135	141	146	152	158	163	169	175	180	186	191	197	203	208	214	220	225	231	237	242	248	254	259	265	270	278	282	287	293	299	304
64	110	116	122	128	134	140	145	151	157	163	169	174	180	186	192	197	204	209	215	221	227	232	238	244	250	256	262	267	273	279	285	291	296	302	308	314
65	114	120	126	132	138	144	150	156	162	168	174	180	186	192	198	204	210	216	222	228	234	240	246	252	258	264	270	276	282	288	294	300	306	312	318	324
66	118	124	130	136	142	148	155	161	167	173	179	186	192	198	204	210	216	223	229	235	241	247	253	260	266	272	278	284	291	297	303	309	315	322	328	334
67	121	127	134	140	146	153	159	166	172	178	185	191	198	204	211	217	223	230	236	242	249	255	261	268	274	280	287	293	299	306	312	319	325	331	338	344
68	125	131	138	144	151	158	164	171	177	184	190	197	203	210	216	223	230	236	243	249	256	262	269	276	282	289	295	302	308	315	322	328	335	341	348	354
69	128	135	142	149	155	162	169	176	182	189	196	203	209	216	223	230	236	243	250	257	263	270	277	284	291	297	304	311	318	324	331	338	345	351	358	365
70	132	139	146	153	160	167	174	181	188	195	202	209	216	222	229	236	243	250	257	264	271	278	285	292	299	306	313	320	327	334	341	348	355	362	369	376
71	136	143	150	157	165	172	179	186	193	200	208	215	222	229	236	243	250	257	265	272	279	286	293	301	308	315	322	329	338	343	351	358	365	372	379	386
72	140	147	154	162	169	177	184	191	199	206	213	221	228	235	242	250	258	265	272	279	287	294	302	309	316	324	331	338	346	353	361	368	375	383	390	397
73	144	151	159	166	174	182	189	197	204	212	219	227	235	242	250	257	265	272	280	288	295	302	310	318	325	333	340	348	355	363	371	378	386	393	401	408
74	148	155	163	171	179	186	194	202	210	218	225	233	241	249	256	264	272	280	287	295	303	311	319	326	334	342	350	358	365	373	381	389	396	404	412	420
75	152	160	168	176	184	192	200	208	216	224	232	240	248	256	264	272	279	287	295	303	311	319	327	335	343	351	359	367	375	383	391	399	407	415	423	431
76	156	164	172	180	189	197	205	213	221	230	238	246	254	263	271	279	287	295	304	312	320	328	336	344	353	361	369	377	385	394	402	410	418	426	435	443

Source: Adapted from *Clinical Guidelines on the Identification, Evaluation, and Treatment of Overweight and Obesity in Adults: The Evidence Report.*

Body Fat Reference:

- Normal: male, 12 to 20 percent; female, 20 to 30 percent
- Borderline: male, 21 to 25 percent; female, 31 to 33 percent
- Obese: male, over 25 percent; female, over 33 percent

This can be measured using several different methods including: skin fold, using a specialized scale (may be available at your weight loss specialist), or immersion in a water chamber with measurement of body density (used mostly at specialized research laboratories).

If you can measure your body fat content, then, by all means, do so. Also keep track of these numbers over time. This becomes especially important when, in addition to diet, a person starts an exercise program and builds up muscle. Some people may find their weight decrease initially as a result of a successful diet and exercise regimen, and yet despite looking and feeling better, the scale starts to go up while the waist line is going down. That is actually a very good sign. The more muscle tissue you have, the higher the metabolic rate (easier to burn calories), and the easier it is to control the weight.

For those who want to keep track of their (or their child's) weight in relation to age, listed below are sample charts that your healthcare professional is likely using:

Up to 2 years of age: *Length-for-age* and *Weight-for-age* charts for boys and for girls. Using length either in inches or centimeters, go across the graph to the vertical line corresponding with the age of the child. Mark the point where they intersect. The same principle goes for the weight. Length should correspond to weight in terms of percentages they fall under.

For example: a child who is between 50 and 75 percent for length, should be in the 50 to 75 percent for weight. If a child is between 50 and 75 percent for length, but over 95 percent for weight, it is an indicator to pay careful attention.

Another thing to keep in mind is that these marks should be followed over time. Some children may stay within the same percentage range as they grow, while others may go either up or down. For instance, a child who starts at 50 percent for both length and weight should stay at or about 50 percent as they grow and develop. Any major change in the pattern is an indicator to touch base with your child's healthcare provider.

Over 2 years of age: BMI-for-age graphs should be used. First calculate the BMI using weight and height (see formulas for both pounds and kilograms on the charts below); then use the calculated BMI in the BMI-for-age percentile chart.

You may find it interesting that BMI of 22 for a 17-year-old male is about 50 percent (or average). Same BMI of 22 for a 5 year old male, however, is extremely overweight. This may be easily missed if the right graph is not used, or used improperly.

Given the importance of this topic, if you are in doubt or not sure how to use these charts, your healthcare provider will likely be able to help (and should be aware).

Appendices

D. *Children and Adolescents Weight Percentage Graphs*

English Formula:
BMI = Weight in pounds ÷ Height in inches ÷ Height in inches x 703
or
BMI = $lb/inch^2$ x 703

Metric Formula:
BMI = Weight in kilograms ÷ Height in meters ÷ Height in meters
or
BMI = kg/m^2

On the following pages are charts for:

*Girls Length-for-Age and Weight-for-Age Chart (Age 1 day to 36 months)

*Boys Length-for-Age and Weight-for-Age Chart (Age 1 day to 36 months)

*Girls BMI-for-Age Chart (Age 2 years to 20 years)

*Boys BMI-for-Age Chart (Age 2 years to 20 years)

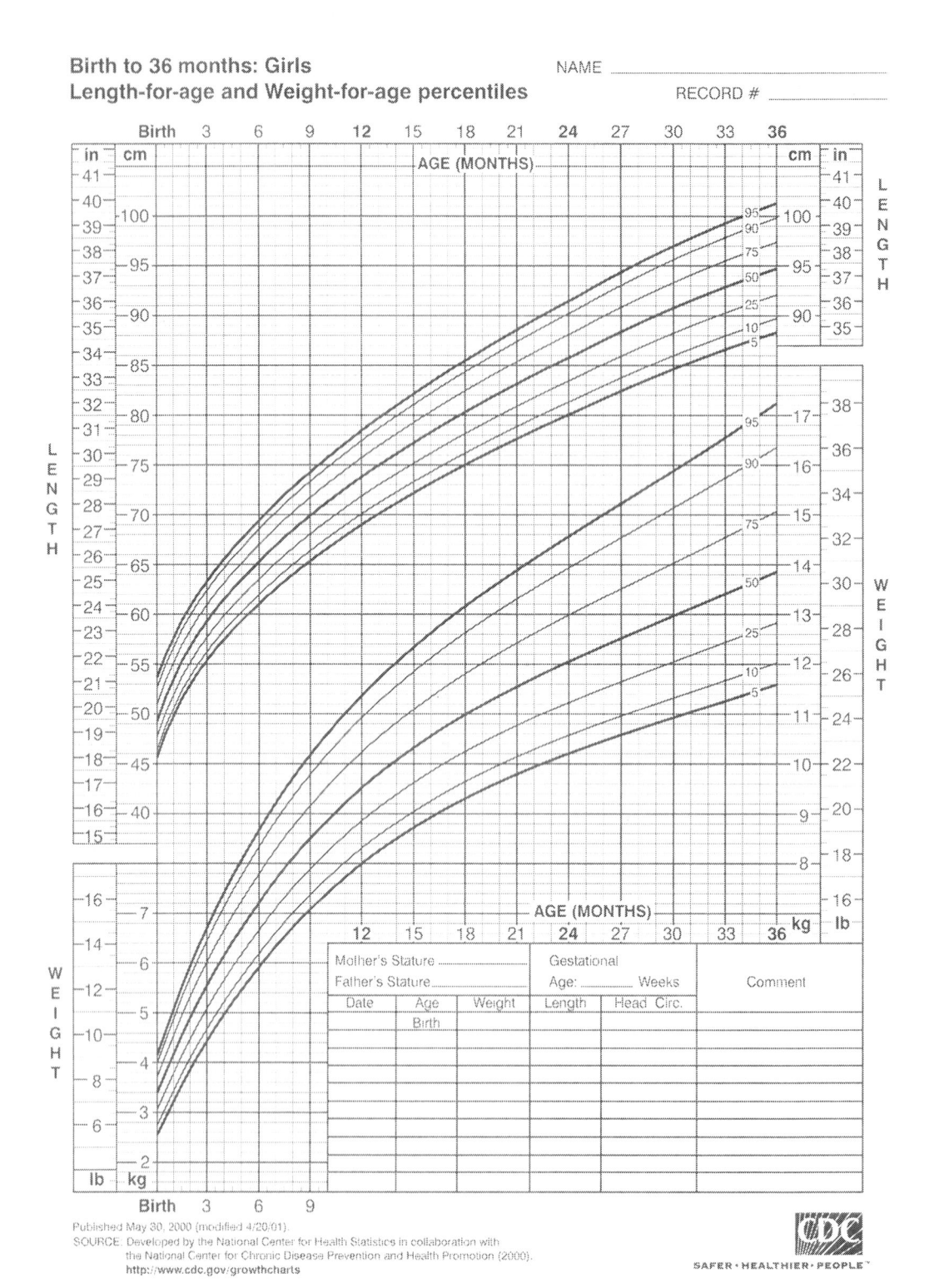

THE POWER PRINCIPLE: MIND-BODY-SPIRIT APPROACH TO ULTIMATE WEIGHT LOSS

Birth to 36 months: Boys
Length-for-age and Weight-for-age percentiles

NAME _____

RECORD # _____

Mother's Stature _____ Gestational
Father's Stature _____ Age: _____ Weeks

Date	Age	Weight	Length	Head Circ.	Comment
Birth					

Published May 30, 2000 (modified 4/20/01).
SOURCE: Developed by the National Center for Health Statistics in collaboration with the National Center for Chronic Disease Prevention and Health Promotion (2000).
http://www.cdc.gov/growthcharts

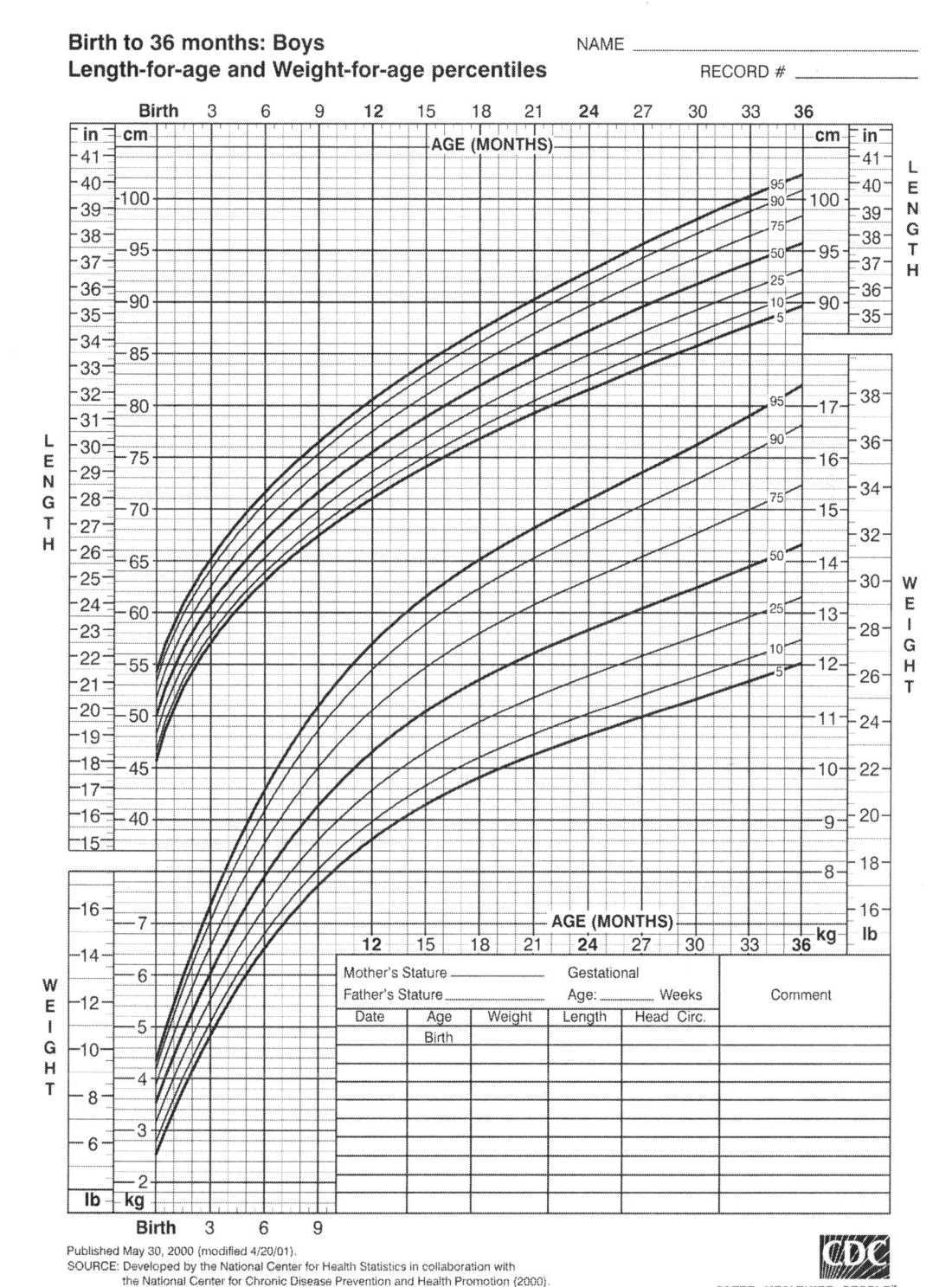

CDC
SAFER·HEALTHIER·PEOPLE™

THE POWER PRINCIPLE: MIND-BODY-SPIRIT APPROACH TO ULTIMATE WEIGHT LOSS

2 to 20 years: Girls
Body mass index-for-age percentiles

NAME _____
RECORD # _____

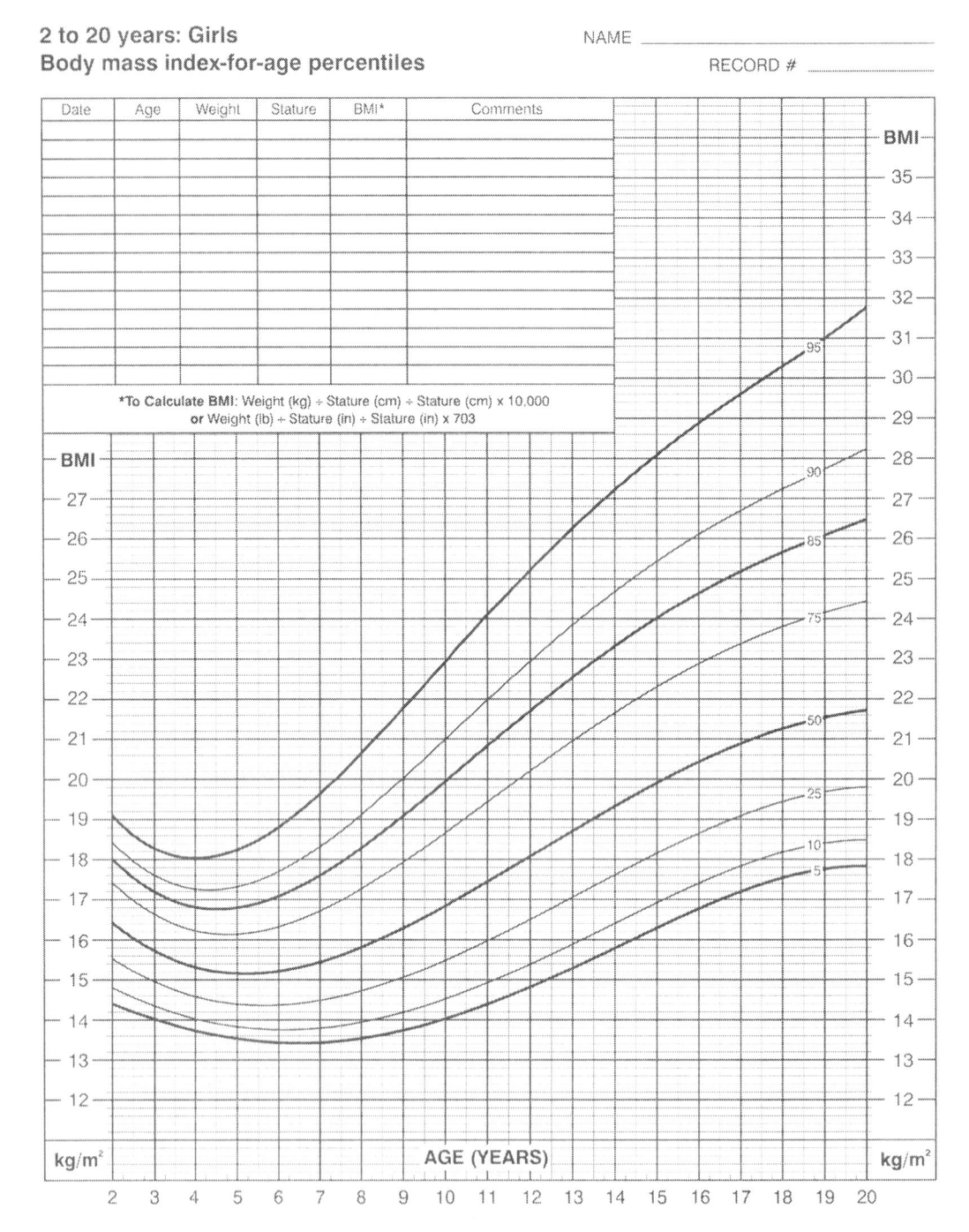

*To Calculate BMI: Weight (kg) ÷ Stature (cm) ÷ Stature (cm) x 10,000
or Weight (lb) ÷ Stature (in) ÷ Stature (in) x 703

AGE (YEARS)

kg/m²

Published May 30, 2000 (modified 10/16/00).
SOURCE: Developed by the National Center for Health Statistics in collaboration with
the National Center for Chronic Disease Prevention and Health Promotion (2000).
http://www.cdc.gov/growthcharts

CDC
SAFER · HEALTHIER · PEOPLE™

134

Appendices

2 to 20 years: Boys
Body mass index-for-age percentiles

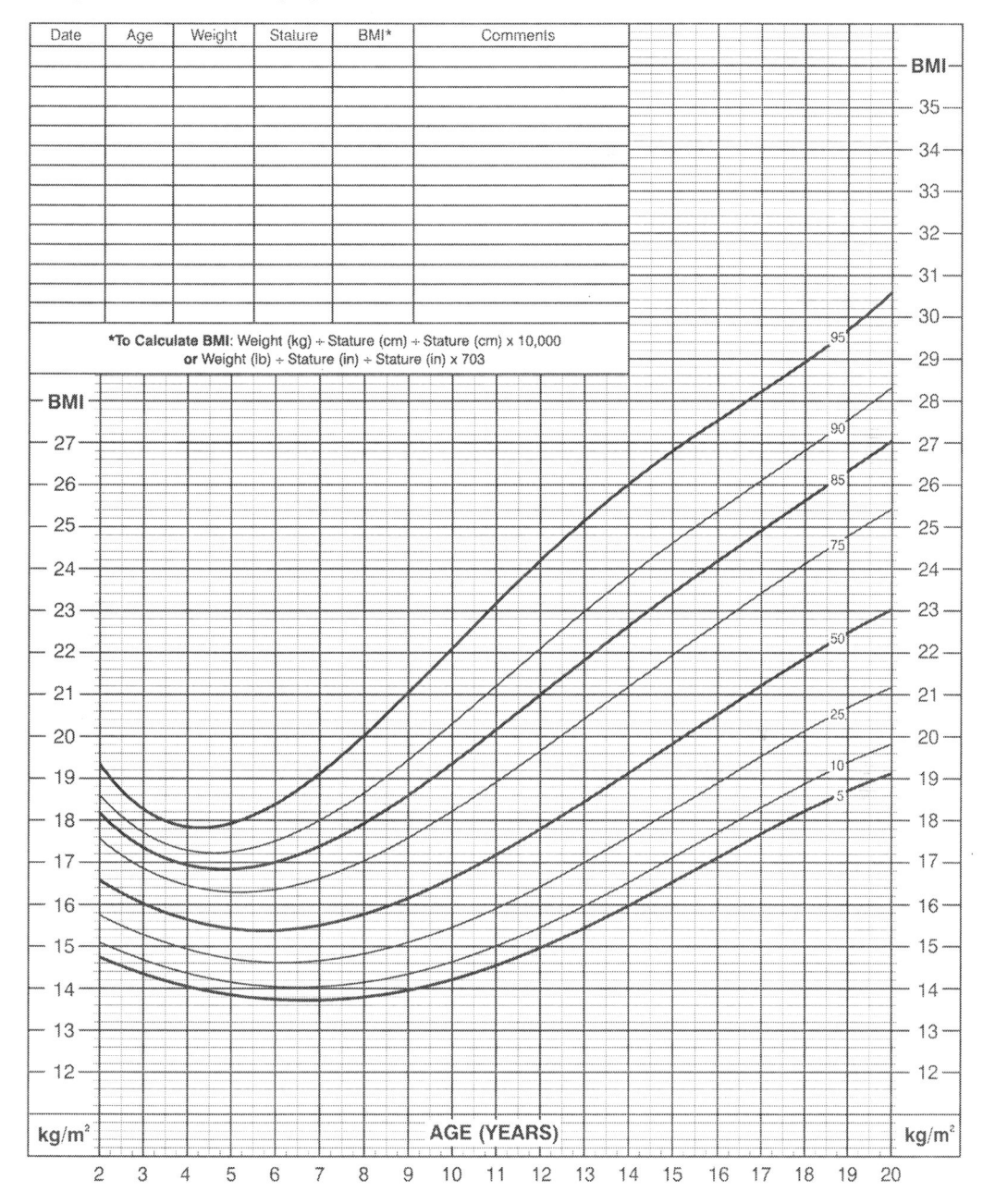

NAME

RECORD #

*To Calculate BMI: Weight (kg) ÷ Stature (cm) ÷ Stature (cm) x 10,000
or Weight (lb) ÷ Stature (in) ÷ Stature (in) x 703

Published May 30, 2000 (modified 10/16/00).
SOURCE: Developed by the National Center for Health Statistics in collaboration with
the National Center for Chronic Disease Prevention and Health Promotion (2000).
http://www.cdc.gov/growthcharts

CDC
SAFER · HEALTHIER · PEOPLE

E. *7-Day Pedometer Weekly Log*

*GOAL: 10,000 or more steps daily

Date: _____

Monday	Tuesday	Wednesday	Thursday	Friday	Saturday	Sunday
_____	_____	_____	_____	_____	_____	_____

Weekly Average: _____

Date: _____

Monday	Tuesday	Wednesday	Thursday	Friday	Saturday	Sunday
_____	_____	_____	_____	_____	_____	_____

Weekly Average: _____

Date: _____

Monday	Tuesday	Wednesday	Thursday	Friday	Saturday	Sunday
_____	_____	_____	_____	_____	_____	_____

Weekly Average: _____

Date: _____

Monday	Tuesday	Wednesday	Thursday	Friday	Saturday	Sunday
_____	_____	_____	_____	_____	_____	_____

Weekly Average: _____

Notes: _____

Goals for the next period (week/month): _____

F. *Sample Daily Food/Exercise Planner:*

Date:_____

My Daily Meal Plan: _____

My Daily Activity Plan: _____

Breakfast:

Lunch:

Dinner:

Other Meals/Snacks:

Activity
Type:
Duration:
Intensity:
Pedometer Steps (10,000 or more goal):

Notes and Observations:

Ideas and Suggestions for Lifestyle and Long-term Changes:

G. Suggested Adult High Protein, Low Carbohydrate, Low Fat Diet Plans

800 Calorie High Protein, Low Carbohydrate, Low Fat Diet

Exchanges for the day:
Protein/Meat/Fish-8 oz
Fruit-1 to 4 servings
Vegetables: 4 or more servings
Discretionary/oils: 20 calories

Water 64 oz per day
Multivitamin (general)
Fiber Supplement as needed for constipation
Fish Oil or Omega-3 and Omega-6 supplement

Suggested division of food:
Breakfast:
Protein: Cottage cheese 3-4 oz or 2 eggs and turkey bacon
Fruit: 1 serving of blueberries or equivalent
Vegetables: as desired
Other:

Lunch:
Protein: chicken or fish 2-3 oz
Fruit: 1 (as desert)
Vegetables: 2 or more servings
Other:

Snacks:
Protein: 0
Fruit: 1-2
Vegetables: as desired
Other:

Dinner:
Protein: chicken/ fish or another equivalent 2-3 oz
Fruit: 1 (as desert)
Vegetables: 2 or more servings
Other:

Exercise/ Activity:
Aerobic:
Resistance:
Stretching:
Pedometer Steps (10,000 or more steps goal per day):

1000 Calorie High Protein, Low Carbohydrate, Low Fat Diet

Exchanges for the day:

Protein/Meat/Fish-11 oz
Fruit-1 to 4 servings
Vegetables: 4 or more servings
Discretionary/oils: 40 calories

Water 64 oz per day
Multivitamin (general)
Fiber Supplement as needed for constipation
Fish Oil or Omega-3 and Omega-6 supplement

Suggested division of food:

Breakfast:
Protein: Cottage cheese 3-4 oz or 2 eggs and turkey bacon
Fruit: 1 serving of blueberries or equivalent
Vegetables: as desired
Other:

Lunch:
Protein: chicken or fish 3-4 oz
Fruit: 1 (as desert)
Vegetables: 2 or more servings
Other:

Snacks:
Protein: 0
Fruit: 1-2
Vegetables: as desired
Other:

Dinner:
Protein: chicken/ fish or another equivalent 4-5 oz
Fruit: 1 (as desert)
Vegetables: 2 or more servings
Other:

Exercise/ Activity:
Aerobic:
Resistance:
Stretching:
Pedometer Steps (10,000 or more steps goal per day):

1200 Calorie High Protein, Low Carbohydrate, Low Fat Diet

Exchanges for the day:

Protein/Meat/Fish-14 oz
Fruit-1 to 4 servings
Vegetables: 4 or more servings
Discretionary/oils: 80 calories

Water 64 oz per day
Multivitamin (general)
Fiber Supplement as needed for constipation
Fish Oil or Omega-3 and Omega-6 supplement

Suggested division of food:

Breakfast:
Protein: Cottage cheese 3-4 oz or 2 eggs and turkey bacon
Fruit: 1 serving of blueberries or equivalent
Vegetables: as desired
Other:

Lunch:
Protein: chicken or fish 4-5 oz
Fruit: 1 (as desert)
Vegetables: 2 or more servings
Other:

Snacks:
Protein: 0
Fruit: 1-2
Vegetables: as desired
Other:

Dinner:
Protein: chicken/ fish or another equivalent 6-7 oz
Fruit: 1 (as desert)
Vegetables: 2 or more servings
Other:

Exercise/ Activity:
Aerobic:
Resistance:
Stretching:
Pedometer Steps (10,000 or more steps goal per day):

1400 Calorie High Protein, Low Carbohydrate, Low Fat Diet

Exchanges for the day:

Protein/Meat/Fish-15 oz
Fruit-1 to 5 servings
Vegetables: 6 or more servings
Discretionary/oils: 120 calories

Water 64 oz per day
Multivitamin (general)
Fiber Supplement as needed for constipation
Fish Oil or Omega-3 and Omega-6 supplement

Suggested division of food:

Breakfast:
Protein: Cottage cheese 3-4 oz or 2 eggs and turkey bacon
Fruit: 1 serving of blueberries or equivalent
Vegetables: as desired
Other:

Lunch:
Protein: chicken or fish 5-6 oz
Fruit: 1 (as desert)
Vegetables: 2 or more servings
Other:

Snacks:
Protein: 0
Fruit: 2-3
Vegetables: as desired
Other:

Dinner:
Protein: chicken/ fish or another equivalent 6-7 oz
Fruit: 1 (as desert)
Vegetables: 2 or more servings
Other:

Exercise/ Activity:
Aerobic:
Resistance:
Stretching:
Pedometer Steps (10,000 or more steps goal per day):

1500 Calorie High Protein, Low Carbohydrate, Low Fat Diet

Exchanges for the day:

Protein/Meat/Fish-16 oz
Fruit-1 to 5 servings
Vegetables: 6 or more servings
Discretionary/oils: 160 calories

Water 64 oz per day
Multivitamin (general)
Fiber Supplement as needed for constipation
Fish Oil or Omega-3 and Omega-6 supplement

Suggested division of food:

Breakfast:
Protein: Cottage cheese 3-4 oz or 2 eggs and turkey bacon
Fruit: 1 serving of blueberries or equivalent
Vegetables: as desired
Other:

Lunch:
Protein: chicken or fish 6-7 oz
Fruit: 1 (as desert)
Vegetables: 2 or more servings
Other:

Snacks:
Protein: 0
Fruit: 2-3
Vegetables: as desired
Other:

Dinner:
Protein: chicken/ fish or another equivalent 6-7 oz
Fruit: 1 (as desert)
Vegetables: 2 or more servings
Other:

Exercise/ Activity:
Aerobic:
Resistance:
Stretching:
Pedometer Steps (10,000 or more steps goal per day):

H. Suggested Adult Balanced Diet Plans

800 Calorie Balanced Diet

Exchanges for the day:

Protein/Meat-8
Starch/Carbs-2 or less
Fruit-1
Fat-1 (1 tsp)
Veg-4 or more
Dairy/Milk-0 or less

Water 64 oz per day
Multivitamin (general)
Fish Oil or Omega-3 and Omega-6 supplement
Fiber Supplement as needed for constipation

Suggested division of food:

Breakfast:
Prot-1
Starch-0

Lunch:
Prot-3
Starch-0
Veg-2

Mid-PM Snack:
Dairy-0
Fruit-1

Dinner:
Prot-4
Starch-2
Veg-2
Fat-1

Dessert:
Dairy-0
Fruit-1

Appendices

Exercise/ Activity:
Aerobic:
Resistance:
Stretching:
Pedometer Steps (10,000 or more steps goal per day):

EXAMPLE OF 800 CALORIE Balanced DIET

BREAKFAST:
1 egg or 2 egg whites

LUNCH:
3 OZ LOW SALT TURKEY BREAST
2 CUPS LETTUCE WITH 1 TBS FAT FREE DRESSING

MID-PM SNACK:
1 APPLE

DINNER:
4 OZ CHICKEN BREAST
1 SMALL BAKED SWEET POTATOE
WITH 1 TSP BUTTER
1 CUP GREEN BEANS
1 LARGE SALAD WITH 1 TBS FAT FREE DRESSING

DESSERT:
1 CUP BLUEBERRIES

1000 Calorie Balanced Diet

Exchanges for the day:

Protein/Meat-8
Starch/Carbs-3 or less
Fruit-2
Fat-1 (1 tsp)
Veg-4 or more
Dairy/Milk-1 or less

Water 64 oz per day
Multivitamin (general)

Fish Oil or Omega-3 and Omega-6 supplement
Fiber Supplement as needed for constipation

Suggested division of food:

Breakfast:
Prot-1
Starch-1

Lunch:
Prot-3
Starch-0
Veg-2

Mid-PM Snack:
Dairy-1
Fruit-1

Dinner:
Prot-4
Starch-2
Veg-2
Fat-1

Dessert:
Dairy-0
Fruit-1

Exercise/ Activity:
Aerobic:
Resistance:
Stretching:
Pedometer Steps (10,000 or more steps goal per day):

EXAMPLE OF 1200 CALORIE Balanced DIET

BREAKFAST:
1 egg
1 slice high fiber bread with 1 tbs all fruit spread

LUNCH:
3 OZ LOW SALT TURKEY BREAST

2 CUPS LETTUCE WITH 1 TBS FAT FREE DRESSING

MID-PM SNACK:
1 APPLE
1 CUP YOGURT

DINNER:
4 OZ CHICKEN BREAST
1 SMALL BAKED SWEET POTATOE
WITH 1 TSP BUTTER
1 CUP GREEN BEANS
1 LARGE SALAD WITH 1 TBS FAT FREE DRESSING

DESSERT:
1 CUP BLUEBERRIES

1200 Calorie Balanced Diet

Exchanges for the day:

Protein/Meat-8
Starch/Carbs-4 or less
Fruit-2
Fat-1 (1 tsp)
Veg-4 or more
Dairy/Milk-2 or less

Water 64 oz per day
Multivitamin (general)
Fish Oil or Omega-3 and Omega-6 supplement
Fiber Supplement as needed for constipation

Suggested division of food:

Breakfast:
Prot-1
Starch-1

Lunch:
Prot-3
Starch-1
Veg-2

Mid-PM Snack:
Dairy-1
Fruit-1

Dinner:
Prot-4
Starch-2
Veg-2
Fat-1

Dessert:
Dairy-1
Fruit-1

Exercise/ Activity:
Aerobic:
Resistance:
Stretching:
Pedometer Steps (10,000 or more steps goal per day):

EXAMPLE OF 1200 CALORIE Balanced DIET

BREAKFAST:
1 egg
1 slice high fiber bread with 1 tbs all fruit spread

LUNCH:
3 OZ LOW SALT TURKEY BREAST
2 CUPS LETTUCE WITH 1 TBS FAT FREE DRESSING

MID-PM SNACK:
1 APPLE
1 CUP YOGURT

DINNER:
4 OZ CHICKEN BREAST
1 SMALL BAKED SWEET POTATOE
WITH 1 TSP BUTTER
1 CUP GREEN BEANS
1 LARGE SALAD WITH 1 TBS FAT FREE DRESSING

DESSERT:
8 OZ SKIM MILK
1 CUP BLUEBERRIES

1400 Calorie Balanced Diet

Exchanges for the day:

Protein/Meat-9
Starch/Carbs-4 or less
Fruit-up to 5
Fat-1 (1 tsp)
Veg-5 or more
Dairy/Milk-2 or less

Water 64 oz per day
Multivitamin (general)
Fish oil or Omega-3 and Omega-6 supplementation
Fiber Supplement as needed for constipation

Suggested division of food:

<u>Breakfast</u>:
Prot-2
Starch-1

<u>Lunch</u>:
Prot-3
Starch-1
Veg-2

<u>Mid-PM Snack</u>:
Dairy-1
Fruit-2

<u>Dinner</u>:
Prot-4
Starch-2
Veg-3
Fat-1
Fruit-1

Dessert:
Dairy-1
Fruit-1

Exercise/ Activity:
Aerobic:
Resistance:
Stretching:
Pedometer Steps (10,000 or more steps goal per day):

EXAMPLE OF 1200 CALORIE Balanced DIET

BREAKFAST:
2 eggs
1 slice high fiber bread with 1 tbs all fruit spread

LUNCH:
3 OZ LOW SALT TURKEY BREAST
3 CUPS LETTUCE WITH 1 TBS FAT FREE DRESSING

MID-PM SNACK:
2 Apples
1 CUP YOGURT

DINNER:
4 OZ CHICKEN BREAST
1 SMALL BAKED SWEET POTATOE
WITH 1 TSP BUTTER
1 CUP GREEN BEANS
1 LARGE SALAD WITH 1 TBS FAT FREE DRESSING

DESSERT:
8 OZ SKIM MILK
1 CUP BLUEBERRIES

1500 Calorie Balanced Diet

Exchanges for the day:

Protein/Meat-10
Starch/Carbs-4 or less
Fruit-up to 4

Fat-2 (1 tsp)
Veg-6 or more
Dairy/Milk-2 or less

Water 64 oz per day
Multivitamin (general)
Fish Oil or Omega-3 and Omega-6 supplement
Fiber Supplement as needed for constipation

Suggested division of food:

<u>Breakfast</u>:
Prot-2
Starch-0

<u>Lunch</u>:
Prot-4
Starch-2
Veg-2

<u>Mid-PM Snack</u>:
Dairy-1
Fruit-2

<u>Dinner</u>:
Prot-4
Starch-2
Veg-4
Fat-2
Fruit-1

<u>Dessert</u>:
Dairy-1
Fruit-1

<u>Exercise/ Activity</u>:
Aerobic:
Resistance:
Stretching:
Pedometer Steps (10,000 or more steps goal per day):

EXAMPLE OF 1500 CALORIE Balanced DIET

BREAKFAST:
2 eggs

LUNCH:
4 OZ LOW SALT TURKEY BREAST
2 CUPS LETTUCE WITH 1 TBS FAT FREE DRESSING
2 Slices of whole wheat bread

MID-PM SNACK:
2 Apples
1 CUP YOGURT

DINNER:
4 OZ CHICKEN BREAST
2 SMALL BAKED SWEET POTATOE
WITH 2 TSP BUTTER
2 CUP GREEN BEANS
1 LARGE SALAD WITH 1 TBS FAT FREE DRESSING
1 serving of blueberries

DESSERT:
8 OZ SKIM MILK
1 CUP BLUEBERRIES

I. Suggested Adult Maintenance Plans

1600 Calorie Balanced Diet

Exchanges for the day:

Protein/Meat-10
Starch/Carbs-5 or less
Fruit-up to 4
Fat-2 (1 tsp)
Veg-6 or more
Dairy/Milk-2 or less

Water 64 oz per day
Multivitamin (general)
Fish Oil or Omega-3 and Omega-6
Fiber Supplement as needed for constipation

Suggested division of food:

<u>Breakfast</u>:
Prot-2
Starch-1

<u>Lunch</u>:
Prot-4
Starch-2
Veg-2

<u>Mid-PM Snack</u>:
Dairy-1
Fruit-2

<u>Dinner</u>:
Prot-4
Starch-2
Veg-4
Fat-2
Fruit-1

<u>Dessert</u>:
Dairy-1
Fruit-1

Exercise/ Activity:
Aerobic:
Resistance:
Stretching:
Pedometer Steps (10,000 or more steps goal per day):

EXAMPLE OF 1600 CALORIE Balanced DIET

BREAKFAST:
2 eggs
1 slice high fiber bread with 1 tbs all fruit spread

LUNCH:
4 OZ LOW SALT TURKEY BREAST
2 CUPS LETTUCE WITH 1 TBS FAT FREE DRESSING
2 Slices of whole wheat bread

MID-PM SNACK:
2 Apples
1 CUP YOGURT

DINNER:
4 OZ CHICKEN BREAST
2 SMALL BAKED SWEET POTATOE
WITH 2 TSP BUTTER
2 CUP GREEN BEANS
1 LARGE SALAD WITH 1 TBS FAT FREE DRESSING
1 serving of blueberries

DESSERT:
8 OZ SKIM MILK
1 CUP BLUEBERRIES

1800 Calorie Balanced Diet

Exchanges for the day:

Protein/Meat-12
Starch/Carbs-5 or less
Fruit-up to 5
Fat-2 (1 tsp)
Veg-7 or more
Dairy/Milk-2 or less

Water 64 oz per day
Multivitamin (general)
Fish Oil or Omega-3 and Omega-6 supplement
Fiber Supplement as needed for constipation

Suggested division of food:

<u>Breakfast</u>:
Prot-2
Starch-1

<u>Lunch</u>:
Prot-5
Starch-2
Veg-2

<u>Mid-PM Snack</u>:
Dairy-1
Fruit-2

<u>Dinner</u>:
Prot-5
Starch-2
Veg-4
Fat-2
Fruit-2

<u>Dessert</u>:
Dairy-1
Fruit-1

<u>Exercise/ Activity</u>:
Aerobic:
Resistance:
Stretching:
Pedometer Steps (10,000 or more steps goal per day):

EXAMPLE OF 1800 CALORIE Balanced DIET

BREAKFAST:
2 eggs
1 slice high fiber bread with 1 tbs all fruit spread

LUNCH:
5 OZ LOW SALT TURKEY BREAST
2 CUPS LETTUCE WITH 1 TBS FAT FREE DRESSING
2 Slices of whole wheat bread or 2 exchanges of rice or pasta

MID-PM SNACK:
2 Apples
1 CUP YOGURT

DINNER:
5 OZ CHICKEN BREAST
2 SMALL BAKED SWEET POTATOE
WITH 2 TSP BUTTER
2 CUP GREEN BEANS
1 LARGE SALAD WITH 1 TBS FAT FREE DRESSING
2 servings of blueberries

DESSERT:
8 OZ SKIM MILK
1 CUP BLUEBERRIES

2000 Calorie Balanced Diet

Exchanges for the day:
Protein/Meat-14
Starch/Carbs-5 or less
Fruit-up to 5
Fat-4 (1 tsp)
Veg-7 or more
Dairy/Milk-2 or less

Water 64 oz per day
Multivitamin (general)
Fish Oil or Omega-3 and Omega-6 supplement
Fiber Supplement as needed for constipation

Suggested division of food:

<u>Breakfast</u>:
Prot-2
Starch-1

Lunch:
Prot-6
Starch-2
Veg-2
Fat-2

Mid-PM Snack:
Dairy-1
Fruit-2

Dinner:
Prot-6
Starch-2
Veg-4
Fat-2
Fruit-2

Dessert:
Dairy-1
Fruit-1

Exercise/ Activity:
Aerobic:
Resistance:
Stretching:
Pedometer Steps (10,000 or more steps goal per day):

EXAMPLE OF 2000 CALORIE Balanced DIET

BREAKFAST:
2 eggs
1 slice high fiber bread with 1 tbs all fruit spread

LUNCH:
6 OZ LOW SALT TURKEY BREAST
2 CUPS LETTUCE WITH 1 TBS FAT FREE DRESSING
2 Slices of whole wheat bread or 2 exchanges of rice or pasta
2 servings of butter or equivalent

MID-PM SNACK:
2 Apples
1 CUP YOGURT

DINNER:
6 OZ CHICKEN BREAST
2 SMALL BAKED SWEET POTATOE
WITH 2 TSP BUTTER
2 CUP GREEN BEANS
1 LARGE SALAD WITH 1 TBS FAT FREE DRESSING
2 servings of blueberries

DESSERT:
8 OZ SKIM MILK
1 CUP BLUEBERRIES

2200 Calorie Balanced Diet

Exchanges for the day:
Protein/Meat-15
Starch/Carbs-5 or less
Fruit-up to 5
Fat-5 (1 tsp)
Veg-7 or more
Dairy/Milk-3 or less

Water 64 oz per day
Multivitamin (general)
Fish Oil or Omega-3 and Omega-6 supplement
Fiber Supplement as needed for constipation

Suggested division of food:

Breakfast:
Prot-2
Starch-1

Lunch:
Prot-7
Starch-2
Veg-2
Fat-2

Mid-PM Snack:
Dairy-2
Fruit-2

<u>Dinner</u>:
Prot-6
Starch-2
Veg-4
Fat-3
Fruit-2

<u>Dessert</u>:
Dairy-1
Fruit-1

<u>Exercise/ Activity</u>:
Aerobic:
Resistance:
Stretching:
Pedometer Steps (10,000 or more steps goal per day):

EXAMPLE OF 2200 CALORIE Balanced DIET

BREAKFAST:
2 eggs
1 slice high fiber bread with 1 tbs all fruit spread

LUNCH:
7 OZ LOW SALT TURKEY BREAST
2 CUPS LETTUCE WITH 1 TBS FAT FREE DRESSING
2 Slices of whole wheat bread or 2 exchanges of rice or pasta
2 servings of butter or equivalent

MID-PM SNACK:
2 Apples
2 CUP YOGURT

DINNER:
6 OZ CHICKEN BREAST
2 SMALL BAKED SWEET POTATOE
WITH 3 TSP BUTTER
2 CUP GREEN BEANS
1 LARGE SALAD WITH 1 TBS FAT FREE DRESSING
2 servings of blueberries

DESSERT:
8 OZ SKIM MILK
1 CUP BLUEBERRIES

2400 Calorie Balanced Diet

Exchanges for the day:
Protein/Meat-17
Starch/Carbs-6 or less
Fruit-up to 5
Fat-5 (1 tsp)
Veg-7 or more
Dairy/Milk-4 or less

Water 64 oz per day
Multivitamin (general)
Fish Oil or Omega-3 and Omega-6 supplement
Fiber Supplement as needed for constipation

Suggested division of food:
<u>Breakfast</u>:
Prot-2
Starch-1
Dairy-1

<u>Lunch</u>:
Prot-8
Starch-2
Veg-2
Fat-2

<u>Mid-PM Snack</u>:
Dairy-2
Fruit-2

<u>Dinner</u>:
Prot-6
Starch-3
Veg-4
Fat-3
Fruit-2

Dessert:
Dairy-1
Fruit-1

Exercise/ Activity:
Aerobic:
Resistance:
Stretching:
Pedometer Steps (10,000 or more steps goal per day):

EXAMPLE OF 2400 CALORIE Balanced DIET

BREAKFAST:
2 eggs
1 slice high fiber bread with 1 tbs all fruit spread
1 Yogurt or another dairy equivalent

LUNCH:
8 OZ LOW SALT TURKEY BREAST
2 CUPS LETTUCE WITH 1 TBS FAT FREE DRESSING
2 Slices of whole wheat bread or 2 exchanges of rice or pasta
2 servings of butter or equivalent

MID-PM SNACK:
2 Apples
2 CUP YOGURT

DINNER:
6 OZ CHICKEN BREAST
3 SMALL BAKED SWEET POTATOE or 3 servings of whole grain pasta or rice
WITH 3 TSP BUTTER
2 CUP GREEN BEANS
1 LARGE SALAD WITH 1 TBS FAT FREE DRESSING
2 servings of blueberries

DESSERT:
8 OZ SKIM MILK or 1 dairy equivalent
1 CUP BLUEBERRIES

2600 Calorie Balanced Diet

Exchanges for the day:
Protein/Meat-18
Starch/Carbs-7 or less
Fruit-up to 5
Fat-7 (1 tsp)
Veg-8 or more
Dairy/Milk-4 or less

Water 64 oz per day
Multivitamin (general)
Fiber Supplement as needed for constipation

Suggested division of food:
Breakfast:
Prot-2
Starch-1
Dairy-1

Lunch:
Prot-9
Starch-3
Veg-8
Fat-3

Mid-PM Snack:
Dairy-2
Fruit-2

Dinner:
Prot-6
Starch-3
Veg-4
Fat-4
Fruit-2

Dessert:
Dairy-1
Fruit-1

Exercise/ Activity:
Aerobic:

Resistance:
Stretching:
Pedometer Steps (10,000 or more steps goal per day):

EXAMPLE OF 2600 CALORIE Balanced DIET

BREAKFAST:
2 eggs
1 slice high fiber bread with 1 tbs all fruit spread
1 Yogurt or another dairy equivalent

LUNCH:
9 OZ LOW SALT TURKEY BREAST
3 CUPS LETTUCE WITH 1 TBS FAT FREE DRESSING
3 Slices of whole wheat bread or 3 exchanges of rice or pasta
3 servings of butter or equivalent

MID-PM SNACK:
2 Apples
2 CUP YOGURT

DINNER:
6 OZ CHICKEN BREAST
3 SMALL BAKED SWEET POTATOE or 3 servings of whole grain pasta or rice
WITH 4 TSP BUTTER
2 CUP GREEN BEANS
1 LARGE SALAD WITH 1 TBS FAT FREE DRESSING
2 servings of blueberries

DESSERT:
8 OZ SKIM MILK or 1 dairy equivalent
1 CUP BLUEBERRIES

2800 Calorie Balanced Diet

Exchanges for the day:
Protein/Meat-19
Starch/Carbs-7 or less
Fruit-up to 5
Fat-7 (1 tsp)
Veg-8 or more
Dairy/Milk-4 or less

Water 64 oz per day
Multivitamin (general) and Fish Oil or Omega-3 and Omega-6 supplement
Fiber Supplement as needed for constipation

Suggested division of food:
Breakfast:
Prot-2
Starch-1
Dairy-1

Lunch:
Prot-9
Starch-3
Veg-8
Fat-3

Mid-PM Snack:
Dairy-2
Fruit-2

Dinner:
Prot-7
Starch-3
Veg-4
Fat-4
Fruit-3

Dessert:
Dairy-1
Fruit-1
Fat-2

Exercise/ Activity:
Aerobic:
Resistance:
Stretching:
Pedometer Steps (10,000 or more steps goal per day):

EXAMPLE OF 2800 CALORIE Balanced DIET:

BREAKFAST:
2 eggs

1 slice high fiber bread with 1 tbs all fruit spread
1 Yogurt or another dairy equivalent

LUNCH:
9 OZ LOW SALT TURKEY BREAST
3 CUPS LETTUCE WITH 1 TBS FAT FREE DRESSING
3 Slices of whole wheat bread or 3 exchanges of rice or pasta
3 servings of butter or equivalent

MID-PM SNACK:
2 Apples
2 CUP YOGURT

DINNER:
7 OZ CHICKEN BREAST
3 SMALL BAKED SWEET POTATOE or 3 servings of whole grain pasta or rice
WITH 4 TSP BUTTER
2 CUP GREEN BEANS or equivalent
1 LARGE SALAD WITH 1 TBS FAT FREE DRESSING
3 servings of blueberries or equivalent

DESSERT:
8 OZ SKIM MILK or 1 dairy equivalent
1 CUP BLUEBERRIES
2 serving of nuts or 2 fat equivalents

3000 Calorie Balanced Diet

Exchanges for the day:
Protein/Meat-19
Starch/Carbs-8 or less
Fruit-up to 6
Fat-8 (1 tsp)
Veg-8 or more
Dairy/Milk-5 or less

Water 64 oz per day
Multivitamin (general) and Fish Oil or Omega-3 and Omega-6 supplement
Fiber Supplement as needed for constipation

Suggested division of food:

Breakfast:
Prot-2
Starch-1
Dairy-2

Lunch:
Prot-9
Starch-4
Veg-8
Fat-4

Mid-PM Snack:
Dairy-2
Fruit-2

Dinner:
Prot-7
Starch-3
Veg-4
Fat-4
Fruit-3

Dessert:
Dairy-1
Fruit-1
Fat-2

Exercise/ Activity:
Aerobic:
Resistance:
Stretching:
Pedometer Steps (10,000 or more steps goal per day):

EXAMPLE OF 3000 CALORIE Balanced DIET

BREAKFAST:
2 eggs
1 slice high fiber bread with 1 tbs all fruit spread
2 Yogurt or another dairy equivalent

LUNCH:
9 OZ LOW SALT TURKEY BREAST

3 CUPS LETTUCE WITH 1 TBS FAT FREE DRESSING
4 Slices of whole wheat bread or 4 exchanges of rice or pasta
4 servings of butter or fats/oils equivalent

MID-PM SNACK:
2 Apples
2 CUP YOGURT

DINNER:
7 OZ CHICKEN BREAST
3 SMALL BAKED SWEET POTATOE or 3 servings of whole grain pasta or rice
WITH 4 TSP BUTTER
2 CUP GREEN BEANS or equivalent
1 LARGE SALAD WITH 1 TBS FAT FREE DRESSING
3 servings of blueberries or equivalent

DESSERT:
8 OZ SKIM MILK or 1 dairy equivalent
1 CUP BLUEBERRIES
2 serving of nuts or 2 fat equivalents

3200 Calorie Balanced Diet

Exchanges for the day:
Protein/Meat-20
Starch/Carbs-9 or less
Fruit-up to 6
Fat-8 (1 tsp)
Veg-10 or more
Dairy/Milk-5 or less

Water 64 oz per day
Multivitamin (general) and Fish Oil or Omega-3 and Omega-6 supplement
Fiber Supplement as needed for constipation

Suggested division of food:

<u>Breakfast</u>:
Prot-2
Starch-1
Dairy-2

Lunch:
Prot-9
Starch-4
Veg-8
Fat-4

Mid-PM Snack:
Dairy-2
Fruit-2

Dinner:
Prot-8
Starch-4
Veg-4
Fat-4
Fruit-3

Dessert:
Dairy-1
Fruit-1
Fat-4

Exercise/ Activity:
Aerobic:
Resistance:
Stretching:
Pedometer Steps (10,000 or more steps goal per day):

EXAMPLE OF 3200 CALORIE Balanced DIET

BREAKFAST:
2 eggs
1 slice high fiber bread with 1 tbs all fruit spread
2 Yogurt or another dairy equivalent

LUNCH:
9 OZ LOW SALT TURKEY BREAST
3 CUPS LETTUCE WITH 1 TBS FAT FREE DRESSING
4 Slices of whole wheat bread or 4 exchanges of rice or pasta
4 servings of butter or fats/oils equivalent

MID-PM SNACK:
2 Apples
2 CUP YOGURT

DINNER:
8 OZ CHICKEN BREAST
4 SMALL BAKED SWEET POTATOE or 4 servings of whole grain pasta or rice
WITH 4 TSP BUTTER
2 CUP GREEN BEANS or equivalent
1 LARGE SALAD WITH 1 TBS FAT FREE DRESSING
3 servings of blueberries or equivalent

DESSERT:
8 OZ SKIM MILK or 1 dairy equivalent
1 CUP BLUEBERRIES
4 serving of nuts or 4 fat equivalents

J. Suggested Children and Adolescent Diet Plans:

Pediatric Diet Meal Plans for 2-3 years old (800 Calories)

Grains/Starches: 3 oz or exchanges
Vegetables: 1 cup or exchange
Fruit: 1 cup or exchange
Milk: 2 cups or exchanges
Meat/Meat Equivalents: 2 oz or exchanges
Fats: 3 tsp
Extra calories: up to 40 Cal
Activity: more than 60 minutes extra physical activity per day

<u>**My daily meal and activity plan**</u>
Breakfast:
Grains/Starches:
Vegetables:
Fruit:
Milk:
Meat/Meat Equivalents:
Fats:
Extra calories:

Lunch:
Grains/Starches:
Vegetables:
Fruit:
Milk:
Meat/Meat Equivalents:
Fats:
Extra calories:

Dinner:
Grains/Starches:
Vegetables:
Fruit:
Milk:
Meat/Meat Equivalents:
Fats:
Extra calories:

Snacks:
Grains/Starches:
Vegetables:
Fruit:
Milk:
Meat/Meat Equivalents:

Fats:
Extra calories:

Activity:
Type:
Duration:
Intensity:

Pediatric Diet Meal Plans for 4-8 years old (900-1200 Calories)

Grains/Starches: 3 to 5 oz or exchanges
Vegetables: 1.5 cup or exchange
Fruit: 1 to 1.5 cup or exchange
Milk: 2 cups or exchanges
Meat/Meat Equivalents: 3 to 4 oz or exchanges
Fats: 4 tsp
Extra calories: up to 40 Cal
Activity: more than 60 minutes extra physical activity per day

My daily meal and activity plan
Breakfast:
Grains/Starches:
Vegetables:
Fruit:
Milk:
Meat/Meat Equivalents:
Fats:
Extra calories:

Lunch:
Grains/Starches:
Vegetables:
Fruit:
Milk:
Meat/Meat Equivalents:
Fats:
Extra calories:

Dinner:
Grains/Starches:
Vegetables:
Fruit:
Milk:
Meat/Meat Equivalents:
Fats:
Extra calories:

Snacks:
Grains/Starches:
Vegetables:
Fruit:
Milk:
Meat/Meat Equivalents:
Fats:
Extra calories:

Activity:
Type:
Duration:
Intensity:

Pediatric Diet Meal Plans for over 9 years old (1200-1600 Calories)

Grains/Starches: 3 to 6 oz or exchanges
Vegetables: 2 to 3 cups or exchanges
Fruit: 1.5 to 2 cups or exchanges
Milk: 3 cups or exchanges
Meat/Meat Equivalents: 5 to 6 oz or exchanges
Fats: 5 tsp
Extra calories: up to 40 Cal
Activity: more than 60 minutes extra physical activity per day

My daily meal and activity plan:
Breakfast:
Grains/Starches:
Vegetables:
Fruit:
Milk:
Meat/Meat Equivalents:
Fats:
Extra calories:

Lunch:
Grains/Starches:
Vegetables:
Fruit:
Milk:
Meat/Meat Equivalents:
Fats:
Extra calories:

Dinner:
Grains/Starches:
Vegetables:

Fruit:
Milk:
Meat/Meat Equivalents:
Fats:
Extra calories:

Snacks:
Grains/Starches:
Vegetables:
Fruit:
Milk:
Meat/Meat Equivalents:
Fats:
Extra calories:

Activity:
Type:
Duration:
Intensity:

(Adapted from: http://www.mypyramid.gov)

K. Suggested Children and Adolescent Dietary Maintenance Plans: (Adapted from: http://www.mypyramid.gov)

Pediatric suggested daily meal plans (1000 Calories)
Grains/Starches: 3 oz or exchanges
Vegetables: 1 cup or exchange
Fruit: 1 cup or exchange
Milk: 2 cups or exchanges
Meat/Meat Equivalents: 2 oz or exchanges
Extra calories: up to 165 Cal
Activity: more than 60 minutes extra physical activity per day

My daily meal and activity plan
Breakfast:
Grains/Starches:
Vegetables:
Fruit:
Milk:
Meat/Meat Equivalents:
Extra calories:

Lunch:
Grains/Starches:
Vegetables:
Fruit:
Milk:
Meat/Meat Equivalents:
Extra calories:

Dinner:
Grains/Starches:
Vegetables:
Fruit:
Milk:
Meat/Meat Equivalents:
Extra calories:

Snacks:
Grains/Starches:
Vegetables:
Fruit:
Milk:
Meat/Meat Equivalents:
Extra calories:

Activity:
Type:
Duration:
Intensity:

Pediatric suggested daily meal plans (1200 Calories)

Grains/Starches: 4 oz or exchanges
Vegetables: 1.5 cup or exchange
Fruit: 1 cup or exchange
Milk: 2 cups or exchanges
Meat/Meat Equivalents: 3 oz or exchanges
Extra calories: up to 170 Cal
Activity: more than 60 minutes extra physical activity per day

My daily meal and activity plan
Breakfast:
Grains/Starches:
Vegetables:
Fruit:
Milk:
Meat/Meat Equivalents:
Extra calories:

Lunch:
Grains/Starches:
Vegetables:
Fruit:
Milk:
Meat/Meat Equivalents:
Extra calories:

Dinner:
Grains/Starches:
Vegetables:
Fruit:
Milk:
Meat/Meat Equivalents:
Extra calories:

Snacks:
Grains/Starches:
Vegetables:
Fruit:
Milk:
Meat/Meat Equivalents:
Extra calories:

Activity:
Type:
Duration:
Intensity:

Pediatric suggested daily meal plans (1400 Calories)

Grains/Starches: 5 oz or exchanges
Vegetables: 1.5 cup or exchange
Fruit: 1.5 cup or exchange
Milk: 2 cups or exchanges
Meat/Meat Equivalents: 4 oz or exchanges
Extra calories: up to 170 Cal
Activity: more than 60 minutes extra physical activity per day

My daily meal and activity plan
Breakfast:
Grains/Starches:
Vegetables:
Fruit:
Milk:
Meat/Meat Equivalents:
Extra calories:

Lunch:
Grains/Starches:
Vegetables:
Fruit:
Milk:
Meat/Meat Equivalents:
Extra calories:

Dinner:
Grains/Starches:
Vegetables:
Fruit:
Milk:
Meat/Meat Equivalents:
Extra calories:

Snacks:
Grains/Starches:
Vegetables:
Fruit:
Milk:
Meat/Meat Equivalents:
Extra calories:

Activity:
Type:
Duration:
Intensity:

Pediatric suggested daily meal plans (1600 Calories)

Grains/Starches: 5 oz or exchanges
Vegetables: 2 cup or exchange
Fruit: 1.5 cup or exchange
Milk: 3 cups or exchanges
Meat/Meat Equivalents: 5 oz or exchanges
Extra calories: up to 130 Cal
Activity: more than 60 minutes extra physical activity per day

My daily meal and activity plan
Breakfast:
Grains/Starches:
Vegetables:
Fruit:
Milk:
Meat/Meat Equivalents:
Extra calories:

Lunch:
Grains/Starches:
Vegetables:
Fruit:
Milk:
Meat/Meat Equivalents:
Extra calories:

Dinner:
Grains/Starches:
Vegetables:
Fruit:
Milk:
Meat/Meat Equivalents:
Extra calories:

Snacks:
Grains/Starches:
Vegetables:
Fruit:
Milk:
Meat/Meat Equivalents:
Extra calories:

Activity:
Type:
Duration:
Intensity:

Pediatric suggested daily meal plans (1800 Calories)

Grains/Starches: 6 oz or exchanges
Vegetables: 2.5 cup or exchange
Fruit: 1.5 cup or exchange
Milk: 3 cups or exchanges
Meat/Meat Equivalents: 5 oz or exchanges
Extra calories: up to 195 Cal
Activity: more than 60 minutes extra physical activity per day

My daily meal and activity plan
Breakfast:
Grains/Starches:
Vegetables:
Fruit:
Milk:
Meat/Meat Equivalents:
Extra calories:

Lunch:
Grains/Starches:
Vegetables:
Fruit:
Milk:
Meat/Meat Equivalents:
Extra calories:

Dinner:
Grains/Starches:
Vegetables:
Fruit:
Milk:
Meat/Meat Equivalents:
Extra calories:

Snacks:
Grains/Starches:
Vegetables:
Fruit:
Milk:
Meat/Meat Equivalents:
Extra calories:

Activity:
Type:
Duration:
Intensity:

Pediatric suggested daily meal plans (2000 Calories)

Grains/Starches: 6 oz or exchanges
Vegetables: 2.5 cup or exchange
Fruit: 2 cup or exchange
Milk: 3 cups or exchanges
Meat/Meat Equivalents: 5.5 oz or exchanges
Extra calories: up to 265 Cal
Activity: more than 60 minutes extra physical activity per day

My daily meal and activity plan
Breakfast:
Grains/Starches:
Vegetables:
Fruit:
Milk:
Meat/Meat Equivalents:
Extra calories:

Lunch:
Grains/Starches:
Vegetables:
Fruit:
Milk:
Meat/Meat Equivalents:
Extra calories:

Dinner:
Grains/Starches:
Vegetables:
Fruit:
Milk:
Meat/Meat Equivalents:
Extra calories:

Snacks:
Grains/Starches:
Vegetables:
Fruit:
Milk:
Meat/Meat Equivalents:
Extra calories:

Activity:
Type:
Duration:
Intensity:

Pediatric suggested daily meal plans (2200 Calories)

Grains/Starches: 7 oz or exchanges
Vegetables: 3 cup or exchange
Fruit: 2 cup or exchange
Milk: 3 cups or exchanges
Meat/Meat Equivalents: 6 oz or exchanges
Extra calories: up to 290 Cal
Activity: more than 60 minutes extra physical activity per day

My daily meal and activity plan
Breakfast:
Grains/Starches:
Vegetables:
Fruit:
Milk:
Meat/Meat Equivalents:
Extra calories:

Lunch:
Grains/Starches:
Vegetables:
Fruit:
Milk:
Meat/Meat Equivalents:
Extra calories:

Dinner:
Grains/Starches:
Vegetables:
Fruit:
Milk:
Meat/Meat Equivalents:
Extra calories:

Snacks:
Grains/Starches:
Vegetables:
Fruit:
Milk:
Meat/Meat Equivalents:
Extra calories:

Activity:
Type:
Duration:
Intensity:

Pediatric suggested daily meal plans (2400 Calories)

Grains/Starches: 8 oz or exchanges
Vegetables: 3 cup or exchange
Fruit: 2 cup or exchange
Milk: 3 cups or exchanges
Meat/Meat Equivalents: 6.5 oz or exchanges
Extra calories: up to 360 Cal
Activity: more than 60 minutes extra physical activity per day

My daily meal and activity plan
Breakfast:
Grains/Starches:
Vegetables:
Fruit:
Milk:
Meat/Meat Equivalents:
Extra calories:

Lunch:
Grains/Starches:
Vegetables:
Fruit:
Milk:
Meat/Meat Equivalents:
Extra calories:

Dinner:
Grains/Starches:
Vegetables:
Fruit:
Milk:
Meat/Meat Equivalents:
Extra calories:

Snacks:
Grains/Starches:
Vegetables:
Fruit:
Milk:
Meat/Meat Equivalents:
Extra calories:

Activity:
Type:
Duration:
Intensity:

Pediatric suggested daily meal plans (2600 Calories)

Grains/Starches: 9 oz or exchanges
Vegetables: 3.5 cup or exchange
Fruit: 2 cup or exchange
Milk: 3 cups or exchanges
Meat/Meat Equivalents: 6.5 oz or exchanges
Extra calories: up to 410 Cal
Activity: more than 60 minutes extra physical activity per day

My daily meal and activity plan
Breakfast:
Grains/Starches:
Vegetables:
Fruit:
Milk:
Meat/Meat Equivalents:
Extra calories:

Lunch:
Grains/Starches:
Vegetables:
Fruit:
Milk:
Meat/Meat Equivalents:
Extra calories:

Dinner:
Grains/Starches:
Vegetables:
Fruit:
Milk:
Meat/Meat Equivalents:
Extra calories:

Snacks:
Grains/Starches:
Vegetables:
Fruit:
Milk:
Meat/Meat Equivalents:
Extra calories:

Activity:
Type:
Duration:
Intensity:

Pediatric suggested daily meal plans (2800 Calories)

Grains/Starches: 10 oz or exchanges
Vegetables: 3.5 cup or exchange
Fruit: 2.5 cup or exchange
Milk: 3 cups or exchanges
Meat/Meat Equivalents: 7 oz or exchanges
Extra calories: up to 425 Cal
Activity: more than 60 minutes extra physical activity per day

My daily meal and activity plan
Breakfast:
Grains/Starches:
Vegetables:
Fruit:
Milk:
Meat/Meat Equivalents:
Extra calories:

Lunch:
Grains/Starches:
Vegetables:
Fruit:
Milk:
Meat/Meat Equivalents:
Extra calories:

Dinner:
Grains/Starches:
Vegetables:
Fruit:
Milk:
Meat/Meat Equivalents:
Extra calories:

Snacks:
Grains/Starches:
Vegetables:
Fruit:
Milk:
Meat/Meat Equivalents:
Extra calories:

Activity:
Type:
Duration:
Intensity:

Pediatric suggested daily meal plans (3000 Calories)

Grains/Starches: 10 oz or exchanges
Vegetables: 4 cup or exchange
Fruit: 2.5 cup or exchange
Milk: 3 cups or exchanges
Meat/Meat Equivalents: 7 oz or exchanges
Extra calories: up to 510 Cal
Activity: more than 60 minutes extra physical activity per day

My daily meal and activity plan
Breakfast:
Grains/Starches:
Vegetables:
Fruit:
Milk:
Meat/Meat Equivalents:
Extra calories:

Lunch:
Grains/Starches:
Vegetables:
Fruit:
Milk:
Meat/Meat Equivalents:
Extra calories:

Dinner:
Grains/Starches:
Vegetables:
Fruit:
Milk:
Meat/Meat Equivalents:
Extra calories:

Snacks:
Grains/Starches:
Vegetables:
Fruit:
Milk:
Meat/Meat Equivalents:
Extra calories:

Activity:
Type:
Duration:
Intensity:

Pediatric suggested daily meal plans (3200 Calories)

Grains/Starches: 10 oz or exchanges
Vegetables: 4 cup or exchange
Fruit: 2.5 cup or exchange
Milk: 3 cups or exchanges
Meat/Meat Equivalents: 7 oz or exchanges
Extra calories: up to 650 Cal
Activity: more than 60 minutes extra physical activity per day

My daily meal and activity plan
Breakfast:
Grains/Starches:
Vegetables:
Fruit:
Milk:
Meat/Meat Equivalents:
Extra calories:

Lunch:
Grains/Starches:
Vegetables:
Fruit:
Milk:
Meat/Meat Equivalents:
Extra calories:

Dinner:
Grains/Starches:
Vegetables:
Fruit:
Milk:
Meat/Meat Equivalents:
Extra calories:

Snacks:
Grains/Starches:
Vegetables:
Fruit:
Milk:
Meat/Meat Equivalents:
Extra calories:

Activity:
Type:
Duration:
Intensity:

L. Choosing a Medical Weight Loss Program
(Adapted from: http://win.niddk.nih.gov/publications/choosing.htm)

Gather as much information as you can before deciding to join a program. Professionals working for weight-loss programs should be able to answer these questions:

Does the program offer one-on-one counseling or group classes?

Do you have to follow a specific meal plan or keep food records?

Do you have to purchase special food, drugs, or supplements?

Does the program help you be more physically active, follow a specific physical activity plan, or provide exercise instruction?

Does the program teach you to make positive and healthy behavior changes?

Is the program sensitive to your lifestyle and cultural needs?

What are the staff qualifications?

Who supervises the program?

What type of weight management training, experience, education, and certifications do the staff have?

Do the products or program carry any risks?

Could the recommended drugs or supplements harm your health?

Do participants talk with a doctor?

Does a doctor run the program?

Will the program's doctors work with your personal doctor if you have a medical condition such as high blood pressure or are taking prescribed drugs?

How much does the program cost?

What is the total cost of the program?

Are there other costs, such as weekly attendance fees, food and supplement purchases, etc.?

Are there fees for a follow-up program after you lose weight?

Are there other fees for medical tests?

What results do participants typically have?

How much weight does an average participant lose and how long does he or she keep the weight off?

Does the program offer publications or materials that describe what results participants typically have?

References and Resources

American Society of Bariatric Physicians (www.ASBP.org)

http://www.MyPyramid.GOV

American Dietetic Association (ADA)

http://www.CDC.gov

http://www.Uptodate.com

National Weight Control registry